Beyond the Lit Screen

By

D. L. Hawkins

A *Plan* for PARENTS To Reclaim their Relationship with Their Children Amidst Social Media Addiction

BEYOND THE LIT SCREEN

A PLAN FOR PARENTS TO RECLAIM THEIR RELATIONSHIP WITH THEIR CHILDREN AMIDST SOCIAL MEDIA ADDICTION

D. L. HAWKINS

CONTENTS

INTRODUCTION

In an age dominated by digital connectivity, where the pervasive glow of screens illuminates our lives, the intimate fabric of family relationships is undergoing a profound transformation. This transformation is particularly palpable in households where parents find themselves grappling with the challenge of raising young children and teenagers engrossed in the captivating world of social media. The book at hand is a compass for these parents, a guide through the intricate terrain of modern parenthood, where the incessant pull of digital devices threatens to unravel the very bonds that tie families together.

The ubiquity of smartphones and social media platforms has ushered in an era where attention is a precious commodity, and its scarcity is acutely felt in homes across the globe. For parents, this presents a daunting dilemma: how to foster meaningful connections with their children when the allure of screens is an ever-present distraction. This dilemma is not just a modern inconvenience but a pressing societal issue, with farreaching consequences for familial harmony and the emotional well-being of both parents and their offspring.

As we embark on this exploration, it's crucial to acknowledge the multifaceted nature of the challenge. Parents are not merely contending with the allure of social media; they are contending with the transformation of communication itself. The devices that now seem like extensions of our hands are simultaneously connecting and disconnecting us from one another. In the realm of parenting, this paradox is especially pronounced, as screens become both a bridge and a barrier between generations.

The genesis of this book lies in the lived experiences of countless parents who have found themselves on the precipice of a digital divide, watching as their relationships with their children become strained under the weight of constant connectivity. The narratives that unfold within these pages are not just cautionary tales but invitations to introspection and, ultimately, action. For it is through understanding the root causes of this digital disconnection that parents can begin the journey toward re-establishing genuine connections with their children.

The first chapters of this book delve into the intricacies of the digital landscape that now shapes the world of our children. We explore the psychology behind the allure of social media and the addictive nature of digital platforms. By understanding the forces that captivate young minds, parents can better empathize with their children's struggles to tear themselves away from their screens. It's a delicate dance between acknowledging the appeal of the digital realm and gently guiding our children back into the warmth of real-world interactions.

Simultaneously, this guide navigates the treacherous waters of parental guilt and self-blame. The pervasive narrative that technology is an insurmountable adversary can leave parents feeling powerless, fostering a sense of inadequacy in their ability to bridge the generational gap. We dissect these feelings and offer a nuanced perspective that empowers parents to reclaim their roles as guides in this digital age, rather than passive bystanders.

A central theme throughout the book is the critical importance of communication—both within the family unit and between parents and their children. We explore strategies for initiating meaningful conversations that transcend the surface and delve into the emotions and experiences that shape the lives of young individuals. In a world where digital communication often takes precedence, rediscovering the art of face-to-face conversation becomes an essential tool for parents seeking to rebuild connections.

As we progress through the chapters, we turn our attention to the impact of parental digital habits on the family dynamic. It is not solely the children who are ensnared by the allures of social media; parents, too, find themselves entangled in the web of digital distraction. The book provides practical advice on fostering a healthy balance between the virtual and the real, emphasizing the need for parents to model the behavior they wish to see in their children.

Ultimately, this book is a roadmap for parents seeking to navigate the complex landscape of modern parenting. It offers insights, strategies, and narratives that illuminate the path toward reconnecting with children who have been momentarily lost in the glow of their screens. The stories shared within these pages are not just cautionary tales but blueprints for a future where familial relationships can flourish beyond the confines of the digital divide. As we embark on this journey together, let us rediscover the power of genuine connection, one conversation at a time, and forge stronger bonds that withstand the everchanging tides of technology.

1

UNDERSTANDING SOCIAL MEDIA ADDICTION

THE ADDICTIVE NATURE OF SOCIAL MEDIA

In the digital age, where the allure of social media is omnipresent, understanding the addictive nature of these platforms becomes paramount, particularly when it starts affecting the very fabric of family relationships. This chapter embarks on an exploration of the various elements that contribute to the addictive grip social media can have on individuals, especially parents and their children.

Elements Contributing to Addiction

At the heart of social media addiction lie several compelling elements that act as potent contributors. The constant availability of content, a feature carefully embedded in the design of these platforms, ensures an unending stream of information. Users find themselves ensnared in the never-ending scroll, the next piece of content just a swipe away. This constant influx of information not only feeds curiosity but also taps into the innate human desire for novelty.

Coupled with this is the strategic use of notification systems, a subtle yet powerful tool. The ping of a notification triggers a sense of urgency, creating a Pavlovian response where users feel compelled to check their devices immediately. It's a cleverly designed mechanism that taps into the human psyche, exploiting our instinctual need for social connection and validation.

Another significant contributor to the addictive nature is the gamification of platforms. Social media platforms are not just places for sharing; they are digital playgrounds designed to keep users engaged. Likes, comments, and followers are no longer simple indicators but rather become points in a game where the user constantly seeks validation and recognition. The pursuit of these digital rewards becomes an addictive cycle, influencing behavior and fostering dependency.

Design Strategies Leading to Prolonged Engagement

The architecture of social media platforms is not arbitrary; it's a carefully crafted design aimed at maximizing user engagement. Platforms are intricately developed to encourage extended usage, employing strategies that make disengagement challenging.

Exploring platform design reveals the deliberate orchestration to keep users immersed for prolonged periods. Infinite scrolling, autoplay features, and personalized content recommendations create an environment where the user is enticed to stay connected for longer durations. The psychological impact of these design elements is profound, leading to habitual and, at times, compulsive usage.

In the grand tapestry of social media, social validation stands out as a powerful force. The number of likes, comments, and followers becomes a metric of one's online popularity. This pursuit of approval can become all-consuming, driving users to perpetually seek more engagement. The discussion here dives into how this quest for validation shapes addictive behaviors and its repercussions on familial relationships.

Consequences of Addictive Nature

The addictive nature of social media isn't a mere inconvenience; it has palpable consequences, particularly within the delicate dynamics of parent-child relationships. As users, especially children, fall prey to the seductive features of these platforms, the potential harm to familial bonds becomes evident.

The analysis of addictive features sheds light on their role in contributing to harm in parent-child relationships. As parents find themselves entangled in the web of constant connectivity, the time and attention dedicated to their children diminish. The consequences extend beyond time management issues, permeating into the emotional realm. Children, seeking parental guidance and presence, may feel neglected or second to the alluring glow of the screen.

Furthermore, the psychological impact of addictive social media use on users, particularly children, is a critical facet to explore. Research suggests that prolonged exposure to social media can contribute to feelings of anxiety, depression, and inadequacy. Understanding these consequences is pivotal in comprehending the toll it takes on the mental well-being of both parents and children.

EXCESSIVE SOCIAL MEDIA USE AND ITS IMPACT ON FAMILY DYNAMICS

In the ever-evolving landscape of the digital age, where screens have become omnipresent, the consequences of excessive social media use on family dynamics have emerged as a pressing concern. This exploration delves into the intricacies of how the pervasive nature of social media can create fault lines within the familial fabric.

Increased Conflict

One of the most tangible impacts of excessive social media use is the surge in conflicts within the family unit. As parents and children find themselves entangled in the digital web, clashes often ensue. The examination of these conflicts reveals a myriad of issues stemming from the relentless pull of social media.

Common areas of contention include the perceived neglect that arises when a family member is engrossed in their digital realm. The simple act of scrolling through feeds or responding to notifications can inadvertently communicate a lack of attention or interest in the present moment. This perceived neglect becomes a breeding ground for resentment and frustration, laying the groundwork for conflicts that extend beyond the digital realm.

Moreover, disagreements often arise from disparities in the perceived importance of online interactions. What one family member may see as harmless scrolling, another may interpret as a prioritization of virtual connections over realworld relationships. This misalignment in values and priorities can give rise to heated discussions, challenging the very essence of familial harmony.

Decreased Communication

As conflicts escalate, a natural casualty is often communication. Excessive social media use becomes a silent barrier, impeding the free flow of dialogue within the family. The exploration of this communication breakdown unveils the challenges parents face in fostering open and meaningful conversations.

The very essence of communication relies on presence— both physical and mental. Social media addiction disrupts this fundamental aspect, diverting attention and focus away from the here and now. Parents, engrossed in the digital tapestry, may struggle to fully engage in conversations with their children. The distractions of notifications and the constant urge to check updates can lead to fragmented discussions, where the depth of connection is sacrificed at the altar of virtual engagement.

Challenges further manifest when attempting to discuss sensitive or important matters. The incessant need to check social media can create an environment where serious conversations are overshadowed, delayed, or altogether avoided. The struggle to capture a child's undivided attention becomes a poignant theme, highlighting the hurdles parents face in fostering a space for open and honest communication.

Reduced Quality Time

Perhaps one of the most poignant impacts of excessive social media engagement is the erosion of quality time spent within the family. The analysis of this phenomenon reveals a stark reality— the time parents spend with their children is increasingly compromised by the gravitational pull of social media.

The essence of quality interactions lies in undivided attention and genuine engagement. However, the constant presence of screens disrupts this delicate balance. Parents, succumbing to the allure of digital notifications, may find themselves physically present but emotionally absent during crucial moments with their children. The dinner table, once a sanctuary for shared stories and laughter, transforms into a battleground where screens compete for attention.

The importance of quality interactions in maintaining strong family bonds cannot be overstated. It is within these moments that memories are forged, values are imparted, and a sense of belonging is nurtured. However, the encroachment of social media on these sacred moments jeopardizes the very foundation of familial relationships.

In essence, the impact of excessive social media use on family dynamics is a multi-faceted challenge that extends far beyond the digital realm. It breeds conflict, stifles communication, and robs families of the precious moments that form the tapestry of shared experiences. As we navigate the complexities of the digital age, understanding these impacts becomes crucial for reclaiming the essence of familial connections and fostering a healthy balance between the virtual and the real.

CHALLENGES FACED BY PARENTS IN BALANCING SOCIAL MEDIA USE

In the intricate dance of modern parenting, a pervasive challenge has emerged—the delicate balance between social media engagement and the profound responsibilities of raising children. This exploration delves into the complex landscape where parental duties intersect with the allure of social media, unraveling the challenges faced and the emotional toll it takes on parent-child relationships.

Parental Responsibilities vs. Social Media Engagement

The challenge of balancing parental responsibilities with social media engagement is akin to walking a tightrope suspended between the tangible world of familial duties and the enticing digital realm. This delicate equilibrium requires navigating a landscape where the demands of parenting often clash with the constant pull of social media.

Parents find themselves grappling with the incessant demands of raising children—attending to their needs, guiding them through life's challenges, and creating a nurturing environment. Yet, in this age of perpetual connectivity, the siren call of social media beckons. The exploration of these challenges uncovers the intricate web that parents must navigate to fulfill their responsibilities while resisting the allure of digital distraction.

The sheer accessibility and addictiveness of social media platforms make it a formidable adversary in the battle for parental attention. The need to check notifications, respond to messages, and stay abreast of the digital conversation becomes a relentless undertow, threatening to pull parents away from the present moment. This struggle isn't just a personal one; it has profound implications for the well-being of children.

The potential consequences for children's well-being are multifaceted. As parents find themselves torn between the real and virtual worlds, the risk of neglecting crucial parenting duties looms large. The child seeking guidance may find themselves competing with the glow of a screen for their parent's attention.

This dynamic can foster feelings of insignificance and unimportance, impacting the child's sense of self-worth and emotional well-being.

Impact on Parent-Child Relationships

The emotional toll on parent-child relationships due to parental social media addiction is a poignant facet of this intricate challenge. As parents succumb to the gravitational pull of social media, the repercussions on the delicate threads of familial connection become palpable.

An examination of this impact reveals a landscape fraught with emotional turbulence. Children, in their formative years, crave the presence and guidance of their parents. Yet, when parental attention is hijacked by the digital glow, the emotional void left behind can be profound. Feelings of neglect and detachment become unwelcome companions for children who yearn for the undivided attention of their caregivers.

The emotional toll manifests in various ways. Children may interpret parental preoccupation with social media as a rejection or dismissal of their needs. The emotional availability of parents is compromised, leading to a sense of isolation for the child. The very foundation of trust and security within parentchild relationships is jeopardized, creating fractures that can have enduring consequences.

Insights into these emotional struggles paint a poignant picture of the challenges faced by parents. The quest for connection within the digital realm often comes at the cost of genuine, heartfelt connections with their own children. The toll on parent-child relationships is not just a narrative of personal struggles but a collective societal challenge with far-reaching implications.

In essence, the challenges faced by parents in balancing social media use with their responsibilities are a poignant reflection of the complexities of modern parenting. It is a journey fraught with the constant negotiation of attention, the battle against digital distraction, and the profound impact on the emotional landscape of parent-child relationships. As we navigate this delicate terrain, understanding these challenges is the first step toward reclaiming the essence of parenting—where presence triumphs over the allure of the digital glow.

RECOGNIZING AND ADDRESSING SOCIAL MEDIA ADDICTION

Unveiling the Digital Struggle: Overview of Signs and Symptoms

In the intricate dance of digital connectivity, the emergence of social media addiction casts a shadow on the fabric of relationships. To unravel this phenomenon, we begin by decoding the subtle yet impactful signs that paint a picture of dependency on digital interactions.

Excessive Screen Time The Red Flag

A pivotal sign of social media addiction lies in the hours devoted to screen time. When the boundary between healthy interaction and digital engulfment blurs, it becomes a call to action. The incessant need to check notifications, the constant digital companionship – these are the markers of a struggle that extends beyond habitual use.

Withdrawal Symptoms Unraveling the Emotional and Physical Toll

Social media addiction brings with it a spectrum of withdrawal symptoms, both emotional and physical. From heightened irritability and anxiety to a compulsive need to stay connected, these symptoms offer a glimpse into the emotional turmoil that ensues when the digital lifeline is momentarily severed.

Proactive Steps Early Recognition and Its Importance

The journey towards addressing social media addiction is paved with proactive steps, and the first crucial stride is early recognition. Understanding the significance of spotting these signs in their infancy is not just about acknowledgment but about fortifying the foundation of parent-child relationships and individual well-being.

Open Communication: Building Bridges Through Dialogue

Effective intervention begins with open communication. Establishing a dialogue where concerns can be voiced without judgment creates a safe space for reflection. This empathetic conversation is not just about addressing the symptoms but about understanding the root causes, fostering connection rather than fostering digital isolation.

Setting Clear Boundaries: Frameworks for Responsible Interaction

In the digital realm, setting clear boundaries becomes a compass guiding individuals toward responsible interaction. Rules around social media usage, especially within the family context, create a framework that encourages a balanced approach. Involving children in this process fosters a sense of ownership and understanding, making it a collaborative effort.

Proactive Measures: Allies in the Battle Against Addiction

Embracing proactive measures is essential. Implementing tools and apps that monitor and manage screen time transforms technology into an ally. By providing insights into usage patterns, these tools empower individuals to regain control over their digital habits. It's a collaborative approach where technology becomes a partner in the journey towards balanced interaction.

Children's Well-being Beyond the Individual to the Collective Impact

The impact of social media addiction extends beyond the individual, leaving an indelible mark on the well-being of children—emotionally and academically. As we explore the consequences, we unravel a narrative that echoes in the broader context of the younger generation's experiences in the digital age.

Emotional Landscape: Navigating Neglect and Detachment

Children, exposed to parental social media addiction, traverse an emotional landscape marred by neglect and detachment. The emotional availability of parents, compromised by digital preoccupation, creates a void in the child's world. Addressing this void is not just a personal endeavor but a collective responsibility.

Academic Implications: Distractions and Decline

Academically, the impact is profound. Excessive screen time fueled by social media addiction encroaches upon valuable study hours, leading to a decline in academic performance. The consequences stretch beyond individual achievement, shaping the collective future of a generation grappling with the challenges of the digital era.

Broader Consequences: Shaping Digital DNA

The imprint of parental social media addiction becomes an integral part of the younger generation's digital DNA. It influences how they navigate relationships, balance responsibilities, and engage with the evolving landscape of technology. Recognizing and addressing social media addiction is not just about the individual but about steering the course for the digital generation.

In essence, this exploration is a journey through the intricate tapestry of digital relationships, where recognizing and addressing social media addiction is a call to action—a reminder of the collective impact our digital choices can have on the fabric of family life and the future of the digital generation.

2

THE IMPACT ON PARENT-CHILD RELATIONSHIPS

IMPACT OF SOCIAL MEDIA ADDICTION ON PARENT-CHILD
RELATIONSHIPS

In the intricate dance of modern family life, the looming presence of social media addiction casts a shadow on the delicate fabric of parent-child relationships. This chapter serves as a guide, a compass navigating through the nuanced consequences that excessive social media use can impose on communication, quality time, and the emotional well-being shared between parents and their children.

Setting the Stage: Understanding the Multifaceted Impact

The stage is set, not in the grandeur of a theater but in the intimate spaces of our homes. As we embark on this exploration, it is crucial to grasp the multifaceted nature of social media addiction's impact on parent-child relationships. It is not a single-threaded narrative but a tapestry woven with threads of communication breakdowns, diminished quality time, and the silent erosion of emotional well-being.

Communication Breakdowns The Unseen Cracks

Communication, the lifeblood of any relationship, bears the brunt of social media addiction. As devices become constant companions, conversations become fragmented, interrupted by the incessant buzz of notifications. The once vibrant exchanges between parent and child are replaced by distracted glances at screens, leaving words unspoken and emotions unsurfaced.

The nuances of non-verbal communication, a critical element in understanding each other, often get lost in the digital translation. The subtle shifts in tone, the facial expressions that convey more than words ever could – these nuances fade into the background as the glow of screens takes precedence over face-to-face interaction.

In the realm of social media addiction, miscommunication becomes an unwelcome guest. The distracted mind, preoccupied with the virtual world, struggles to grasp the intricacies of nuanced dialogue. What was intended as a simple conversation can spiral into misunderstandings, creating unseen cracks in the foundation of parent-child relationships.

Quality Time Lost in the Digital Shuffle

Quality time, a currency more valuable than any digital interaction, becomes a casualty of social media addiction. As screens claim more hours of attention, the moments that once defined family bonds slip through the digital cracks. Family dinners turn into silent gatherings, each member engrossed in their digital universe. The shared activities that fostered connection are replaced by solitary scrolling and swiping.

The concept of being physically present yet emotionally absent takes root. The dinner table, once a sacred space for shared stories and laughter, transforms into a silent battleground of screens competing for attention. Quality interactions, the glue that binds families together, are sacrificed at the altar of constant digital engagement.

The consequence is not just a loss of time but a loss of the very essence that makes memories enduring. The laughter that echoed in shared moments, the conversations that wove the narrative of family life – these become fleeting echoes, drowned out by the noise of notifications.

Emotional Well-being Navigating the Silent Storm

Within the silent storm of social media addiction, emotional well-being becomes a casualty. The emotional availability that parents provide, a pillar of support for a child's growth, falters under the weight of digital preoccupation. The child, seeking solace in the reassuring embrace of parental understanding, finds only the cold glow of a screen.

Feelings of neglect and detachment take root, creating a void that no amount of virtual interaction can fill. The emotional landscape, once vibrant with shared experiences and understanding, becomes a barren terrain. The silent cries for attention, masked by the constant hum of social media, echo in the emotional distance that grows within parent-child relationships.

For parents, the realization of this emotional toll becomes a poignant moment of reckoning. The digital preoccupation that seemed innocuous reveals its insidious impact on the emotional well-being of their children. The challenge lies not just in recognizing the storm but in navigating its complexities to rebuild emotional bridges.

The Call to Action: Nurturing Relationships Amidst the Digital Storm

As we navigate the impact of social media addiction on parent-child relationships, it is not a journey devoid of hope. Instead, it serves as a call to action, a rallying cry to reclaim the essence of communication, quality time, and emotional wellbeing within the family dynamic.

Communication Reimagined Bridging the Digital Divide

Rebuilding communication requires a conscious effort to bridge the digital divide. It begins with reclaiming spaces for meaningful conversations, free from the distractions of screens. Family meetings, devoid of devices, become a sacred ritual where everyone has a voice, and each voice is heard.

Active listening becomes the cornerstone. It is not merely hearing words but understanding the emotions that underpin them. Maintaining eye contact, paraphrasing, and asking open-ended questions become tools to dismantle the barriers erected by social media addiction.

Communication, once lost in the digital shuffle, is reimagined as a vibrant tapestry of shared experiences and understanding. It is a deliberate choice to prioritize face-to-face interaction over the virtual clamor, creating a space where words find their resonance.

Quality Time Rediscovered Moments Beyond Screens

Reclaiming quality time is an intentional act of rediscovery. It involves designating tech-free zones or hours, where the focus is solely on shared activities and connections. Family dinners regain their significance as moments of togetherness, free from the intrusion of screens.

Shared activities become the cornerstone of rebuilding connections. Whether it's cooking together, engaging in outdoor adventures, or simply enjoying a board game night, these activities foster a sense of unity that social media addiction had threatened to erode. They are the antidote to the isolation that screens can induce.

Leading by example is paramount. Parents, as the architects of family dynamics, must demonstrate the importance of quality time by actively participating in these moments. It is not just about preaching but about embodying the values of connection and shared experiences.

Emotional Well-being Nurturing the Seeds of Understanding

Addressing the emotional toll requires nurturing the seeds of understanding. It begins with creating an environment where emotions are not silenced by the constant hum of social media but are acknowledged and validated. Parents become not just providers but emotional anchors, fostering an atmosphere of trust and security.

Building emotional bridges involves acknowledging the impact of social media addiction on parent-child relationships. It requires open conversations where both parties express their feelings and concerns. It is a shared journey of understanding the emotional landscape and actively working towards healing the wounds inflicted by digital preoccupation.

In the midst of the digital storm, emotional well-being is not just about soothing the visible wounds but about fortifying the emotional infrastructure of parent-child relationships. It is an ongoing process, requiring patience, empathy, and a commitment to rebuilding what social media addiction sought to dismantle.

COMMUNICATION BREAKDOWNS CAUSED BY EXCESSIVE SCREEN TIME

In the intricate tapestry of family life, communication stands as the loom weaving the threads of connection and understanding. Yet, the pervasive influence of excessive screen time, fueled by the omnipresence of social media, introduces disruptions that threaten to unravel the delicate fabric of meaningful conversations. This exploration delves into the distracting influence of social media and the challenges of miscommunication, examining the toll it takes on both parents and children.

Distracting Influence of Social Media: Unraveling the Threads of Engagement

The glowing screens that beckon from pockets and palms wield a distracting influence that extends beyond mere fascination. Constant social media use becomes a siren call, diverting attention from the present moment and hindering the richness of meaningful conversations within the family.

The allure of social media, with its scrolling feeds and captivating content, competes for the precious currency of attention. Parents, engrossed in the digital tapestry of news, updates, and notifications, find their gaze directed more toward screens than the faces of their children. Children, too, succumb to the captivating allure of virtual worlds, often losing themselves in the quest for likes, comments, and shared content.

The impact on engagement is palpable. Once vibrant conversations, where the nuances of emotions and thoughts were exchanged, now find themselves stifled by the constant intrusion of screens. The distracted mind, ensnared by the digital realm, struggles to invest fully in the art of conversation. The threads of engagement, once tightly woven, begin to unravel under the weight of perpetual distraction.

This unraveling is not a solitary journey; it affects both parents and children. Parents, navigating the dual role of screen time and caregiving, find themselves torn between the demands of the virtual and the tangible. Children, seeking the undivided attention of their parents, encounter a formidable competitor in the glowing screens that demand perpetual acknowledgment.

Challenges of Miscommunication: Navigating the Silence of Screens

Miscommunication, a silent saboteur, emerges as a formidable challenge within the realm of excessive screen time. The lack of face-to-face interaction, a casualty of virtual engagement, spawns a breeding ground for misunderstandings and gaps in comprehension within parent-child conversations.

The subtleties of non-verbal communication, an integral component of understanding, face the risk of extinction. Facial expressions, gestures, and body language, once conduits of nuanced communication, are replaced by the limitations of digital text and emojis. The richness of tone, which conveyed more than words ever could, becomes a casualty of the silent exchanges within messaging apps.

In the absence of face-to-face interaction, the potential for misunderstandings amplifies. Texts devoid of contextual cues, stripped of the emotional nuances that accompany spoken words, become prone to misinterpretation. What was intended as a simple statement takes on varied shades of meaning, subject to the interpretations of the reader.

Children, in their formative years of language acquisition, face the challenge of comprehending the subtleties of communication. The lack of direct interaction hampers the development of crucial skills, leaving them vulnerable to gaps in understanding. Parents, often unaware of the impact of this digital divide, grapple with bridging the chasm of miscommunication that quietly widens.

In the world of screens, the art of listening also undergoes a transformation. The distractions inherent in constant social media use hinder active listening, where the focus is not just on the words spoken but on the emotions and intentions underlying them. Miscommunication, thus, is not solely a result of misunderstood words but a byproduct of a communication landscape disrupted by screens.

Navigating the Silence: Rediscovering the Art of Conversation

As we navigate the challenges of communication breakdowns caused by excessive screen time, the call to action is clear: a rediscovery of the art of conversation. It is an intentional effort to untangle the threads of distraction and miscommunication that threaten the sanctity of parent-child dialogue.

Rediscovering Engagement Amidst Distraction

The distracting influence of social media necessitates a conscious effort to reclaim engagement. Establishing tech-free zones or designated hours within the home becomes a cornerstone for fostering undivided attention. Here, screens are set aside, and the focus shifts entirely to the present moment, creating space for genuine connection.

Leading by example becomes pivotal. Parents, as the architects of family dynamics, must embody the values they seek to instill. By demonstrating a commitment to undistracted engagement, they lay the foundation for children to follow suit. The glow of screens dims in comparison to the luminosity of shared moments and meaningful conversations.

Navigating the Landscape of Miscommunication

Addressing the challenges of miscommunication requires a multifaceted approach. Embracing face-to-face interactions becomes a priority, reinstating the richness of nonverbal cues and the depth of emotional expression. Shared activities that promote direct engagement, whether it's cooking together, playing games, or simply sitting and talking, become catalysts for rebuilding the bridges of understanding.

Parents, cognizant of the impact of digital communication, can also incorporate strategies to enhance comprehension. Encouraging questions, seeking clarifications, and promoting an open dialogue about the challenges posed by virtual communication create an atmosphere where misunderstandings can be addressed proactively.

The Art of Active Listening

Active listening emerges as a powerful tool in navigating the challenges of miscommunication. In a world saturated with digital noise, the deliberate act of tuning in to each other becomes a radical act of connection. Maintaining eye contact, paraphrasing to confirm understanding, and asking open-ended questions create a communication landscape where the art of listening is revived.

This journey toward rediscovering the art of conversation is not devoid of challenges. The allure of screens, deeply ingrained in daily routines, requires a conscious effort to resist. Yet, the rewards are profound – the revival of engagement, the restoration of nuanced communication, and the strengthening of the ties that bind parent and child.

LOSS OF QUALITY TIME AND MEANINGFUL CONNECTIONS

In the intricate dance of family life, the concept of quality time emerges as the heartbeat, the rhythm that sustains the bonds between parents and children. However, the pervasive influence of excessive screen time threatens to disrupt this delicate dance, replacing traditional bonding activities and casting a shadow over the fabric of meaningful connections. Our exploration into this realm takes us through the realms of replaced bonding activities and the negative impact on family relationships.

Replacement of Bonding Activities: The Digital Intrusion

The essence of family bonding often finds its expression in shared activities and experiences. These moments, whether gathered around a dinner table, engaging in outdoor adventures, or simply spending quality time together, contribute to the fabric of familial connections. However, the digital era introduces a formidable contender – the screen – that has the potential to replace these bonding activities.

How Excessive Screen Time Replaces Traditional Bonding Activities

The allure of screens, with their endless scroll of captivating content, competes for the finite resource of time. Family traditions that once revolved around shared activities now face the encroachment of screens, diverting attention and focus. Simple pleasures like family dinners, once a cornerstone of connection, now contend with the glow of devices at the table.

The replacement is subtle yet insidious. Where family outings and adventures once forged lasting memories, the digital realm now beckons with the promise of instant gratification. The shared joy of playing board games or engaging in creative endeavors takes a backseat to the individualized allure of screenbased entertainment. As screens increasingly infiltrate the sacred space of family bonding, the very fabric of these connections begins to unravel.

Consequences When Digital Engagement Supersedes Shared Experiences

The consequences of this digital intrusion are farreaching. The once vibrant tapestry woven with shared experiences now bears the muted hues of solitary screen time. The joy of shared laughter and the warmth of collective moments diminish in the face of isolated engagements with devices.

Family bonds, once fortified through shared activities, face erosion as screens take precedence. Siblings, once companions in play and exploration, find themselves solitary navigators in the digital landscape. Parents, yearning for meaningful connections with their children, are met with the silent glow of screens that replaces the resonance of shared experiences.

This replacement of bonding activities extends beyond the immediate impact on family dynamics. It sets the stage for a gradual shift in priorities, where the digital realm assumes greater significance than the tangible bonds of togetherness. The consequences reverberate not only in the present but echo into the future, shaping the nature of relationships within the family.

Negative Impact on Family Relationships: Strain in the Fabric of Connection

As shared activities diminish and the digital realm asserts its dominance, the negative impact on family relationships becomes increasingly apparent. The loss of quality time, once the cornerstone of familial connections, contributes to a strain in the fabric of these relationships.

The Loss of Quality Time and Its Contribution to Strain

Quality time, defined by the richness of shared moments and genuine connections, serves as the lifeblood of family relationships. When this vital element is compromised by excessive screen time, a strain permeates the very fabric of the familial bond. The once vibrant threads of togetherness begin to fray, leaving behind a tapestry marked by the absence of shared experiences.

The strain manifests in various ways, from increased tension during family interactions to a sense of emotional distance among family members. The nurturing environment that quality time creates, fostering open communication and mutual understanding, succumbs to the digital divide. Conversations become stilted, laden with the weight of unspoken concerns and unmet emotional needs.

Insights into the Potential Erosion of Familial Bonds

The erosion of familial bonds is a gradual process, often unnoticed until the cracks widen. As screens take center stage, interpersonal connections recede into the background. Children, seeking the guidance and companionship of their parents, may find solace in the virtual realms of social media or online communities. Parents, yearning for meaningful interactions with their children, encounter resistance as screens become preferred companions.

The negative impact extends beyond the immediate relationships to permeate the family ecosystem. Sibling bonds, traditionally fortified through shared experiences, face the risk of becoming distant as individualized screen time takes precedence. The once-unifying force of family traditions loses its potency when screens replace the collective engagement that defined these rituals.

The strain in family relationships becomes a silent undercurrent, influencing the emotional well-being of each family member. Children, deprived of the anchoring influence of quality time, may seek validation and connection through online channels. Parents, grappling with the emotional distance created by screens, find themselves navigating uncharted territories of parenting in the digital age.

Navigating the Shadows: Rediscovering Shared Experiences

As we navigate the shadows cast by the loss of quality time and meaningful connections, the path forward invites a rediscovery of shared experiences. It is a journey that requires intentional efforts to reclaim the moments that define family life, a deliberate weaving of the threads of togetherness into the fabric of familial bonds.

Reclaiming Traditions and Shared Activities

The first step toward rediscovery is a return to family traditions and shared activities. Establishing designated times for family dinners, outings, or game nights becomes a deliberate act of prioritizing togetherness. These shared experiences serve as anchors, grounding family members in the richness of connection that screens often seek to replace.

Parents, as architects of family dynamics, play a pivotal role in this rediscovery. Leading by example, they demonstrate the value placed on shared experiences. Whether it's turning off devices during meals, initiating outdoor adventures, or engaging in creative endeavors as a family, parents set the tone for the type of connections they wish to foster.

Fostering Open Communication

The strain in family relationships often finds its antidote in open communication. Creating a safe space for family members to express their thoughts, concerns, and desires becomes paramount. Family meetings, where everyone has a voice, offer a platform for addressing the impact of screens on quality time and interpersonal connections.

Children, in particular, benefit from a dialogue that acknowledges their perspective. Understanding their interests, concerns, and the allure of screens allows parents to tailor shared activities that resonate with the digital generation. In this open exchange, the barriers created by screens begin to crumble, and the potential for genuine connections is rekindled.

Prioritizing Tech-Free Zones and Device-Free Times

In the digital age, the intentional creation of tech-free zones and designated device-free times becomes a revolutionary act. These zones, whether established in shared living spaces or during specific hours of the day, serve as sanctuaries where screens are set aside, and genuine connections take center stage.

Tech-free zones can extend beyond physical spaces to include designated times for shared activities. Whether it's a family movie night, a weekend hike, or a collective cooking session, these moments become sacred in the tapestry of family life. The deliberate choice to disconnect from screens amplifies the value placed on shared experiences, fostering a sense of unity and togetherness.

EFFECTS ON EMOTIONAL WELL-BEING AND MENTAL HEALTH

In the intricate dance of familial relationships, the pervasive influence of social media addiction casts a profound shadow on the emotional well-being and mental health of both parents and children. As we navigate the digital landscape, we unravel the multifaceted impact, exploring the silent struggles that excessive screen time can impose on the delicate fabric of familial connections.

Detrimental Effects of Social Media Addiction

In the silent spaces illuminated by the soft glow of screens, the emotional toll of social media addiction begins to manifest. Excessive screen time, fueled by a constant influx of information and the pursuit of digital validation, becomes a silent contributor to overwhelming feelings of loneliness, anxiety, and depression.

Loneliness in the Digital Age

Within the paradoxical realm of digital connection, the ceaseless scroll can transform the virtual world into an emotional battleground. Parents, entwined in the quest for connection, often find themselves paradoxically fostering disconnection. The curated glimpses into others' lives and the relentless pursuit of validation create a complex emotional landscape.

Anxiety in the Quest for Validation

The digital quest for likes and comments, a seemingly innocuous pursuit, unfolds as a source of anxiety. The unending comparison game and the pressure to conform to digital ideals amplify the emotional struggles within the digital realm. The impact is not confined to individual experiences but reverberates through the shared spaces of home, impacting the very core of familial bonds.

Depression The Silent Struggle

As we delve into the psychological toll, the silent struggle with depression emerges. The emotional resonance of parental battles with social media addiction extends beyond personal experiences, seeping into the collective consciousness of parent-child relationships.

Impact on Children's Development and Self-esteem

Children, in their formative years, navigate a world where the digital and the tangible intertwine seamlessly. The potential long-term consequences of social media addiction on children's emotional development and self-esteem become a focal point of analysis.

Shaping Self-Esteem in the Digital Age

In the gentle unfolding of childhood, where self-esteem takes its formative steps, the digital landscape becomes a shaping force. The quest for digital validation, intertwined with the foundations of self-worth, creates a complex emotional landscape that extends far beyond the immediate.

Implications for Mental Well-being

Insights into the broader implications for children's mental well-being emerge as we traverse the terrain of prolonged exposure to social media. The curated ideals presented online, societal pressures embedded in digital interactions, and constant comparison to digital personas contribute to the intricate dance between the online and offline worlds.

3
SETTING EFFECTIVE BOUNDARIES

SETTING EFFECTIVE BOUNDARIES FOR SOCIAL MEDIA USAGE

As we embark on the journey through the intricate dynamics of familial relationships in the digital age, Chapter 3 serves as a compass, guiding us through the nuanced terrain of setting effective boundaries for social media usage. In a world where screens mediate our interactions, the need for intentional and well-defined boundaries becomes paramount. This chapter is a comprehensive exploration of strategies aimed at mitigating the potential negative impacts of excessive screen time within the family unit.

Navigating the Digital Landscape

The digital landscape has become an integral part of our lives, significantly influencing how families interact. This introduction contextualizes the chapter's focus, acknowledging the pervasive role of social media in shaping family dynamics. It sets the stage for a thoughtful exploration of the strategies that can help families navigate this complex and ever-evolving digital terrain.

Establishing Clear Rules and Expectations

Significance of Specific Rules

At the heart of effective boundary-setting lies the clarity of rules. This section delves into the significance of specificity, emphasizing the need for rules that go beyond merely limiting screen time. Specific rules act as guiding principles, shaping the family's digital engagement in a way that aligns with broader values and goals.

Communicating Rules Effectively

Crafting rules is an art, but conveying them is a nuanced skill. Effective communication of rules is explored in this section, recognizing the importance of articulating the reasons behind the rules. It delves into strategies that foster a dialogue between parents and children, creating an environment of understanding and collaboration.

The Role of Consistency

Consistency is the glue that holds boundaries together. This part of the chapter elucidates how maintaining consistency in the enforcement of rules provides a sense of predictability and security for children. Consistency acts as a stabilizing force, helping children navigate the digital landscape with clarity.

Negotiating Screen Time Limits

Balancing Act Allowing and Limiting

Negotiating screen time limits is a delicate dance between allowing enrichment and instilling healthy boundaries. This section explores strategies for achieving a harmonious balance, ensuring that screen time contributes positively to a child's development without overshadowing other crucial aspects of life.

Involving Children in Decision-Making

Empowering children in decision-making about screen time is a pivotal aspect of effective boundary-setting. Insights are provided on engaging children in conversations about responsible usage, making the negotiation process an educational journey rather than a set of imposed restrictions.

Tips for Effective Implementation

Negotiating screen time limits is an ongoing dialogue that requires adaptability. Practical tips for parents on effective implementation and adjustment as family dynamics evolve are presented. These insights underscore the need for flexibility, recognizing that rules and limits may need refinement as the family navigates the digital landscape together.

Using Parental Control Tools and Apps

The Landscape of Parental Control Tools

The digital age offers a plethora of tools designed to assist parents in managing their children's screen time. This section sheds light on the diverse landscape of parental control tools, exploring their features, benefits, and potential impact on shaping responsible digital habits.

Implementing Tools Effectively

Having tools is one thing; implementing them effectively is another. This part provides insights into seamlessly integrating parental control tools, delving into content filtering, time restrictions, and monitoring features. It emphasizes the symbiotic relationship between tools and the overarching goal of fostering a healthy digital environment.

Navigating Challenges in Implementation

Implementing tools is not without challenges. This section addresses common hurdles and provides strategies for parents to navigate potential roadblocks. It acknowledges the need for parents to stay informed, engaged, and proactive in the use of these tools, ensuring they serve as aids rather than hindrances.

Fostering Digital Well-being

Synthesizing the key takeaways from the exploration of clear rules, negotiated limits, and parental control tools, the conclusion reinforces the interconnectedness of these strategies in fostering digital well-being within the family. It underscores the collective effort required to create a harmonious digital environment that not only addresses challenges but enriches familial connections. As we delve deeper into subsequent chapters, the goal remains clear: to illuminate the path toward a balanced and healthy relationship with technology, ensuring that the digital landscape enhances, rather than detracts from, the fabric of family life.

ESTABLISHING CLEAR RULES AND EXPECTATIONS

Significance of Specific Rules

Clear Guidelines for a Healthier Digital Environment

In today's digitally-driven world, articulating clear and specific rules for social media use within the family is crucial. Emphasizing the importance of such guidelines extends beyond limitations; it creates a framework that cultivates a positive and secure online atmosphere. These rules not only delineate acceptable behavior but also educate children about responsible digital citizenship.

Fostering Responsible Online Conduct

Well-defined rules offer a roadmap for responsible online behavior. By outlining expectations regarding screen time, respectful communication, privacy settings, and content sharing, these guidelines empower children to navigate social media platforms safely. They establish boundaries that minimize confusion, conflicts, and potential risks associated with online interactions.

Communication of Rules to Children

Age-Appropriate Communication Strategies

Effective communication of established rules necessitates tailoring the delivery to the understanding and maturity levels of children. For younger kids, employing visual aids like simple graphics or drawings helps convey basic rules such as sharing only with known individuals and being kind online. As children grow older, engaging in open discussions becomes more impactful, as it allows for an understanding of the rationale behind each rule and the consequences of noncompliance.

Leading by Example

Parents play a pivotal role in modeling the behavior they expect from their children. Demonstrating responsible online conduct and discussing the reasons behind established rules creates an environment where children understand the importance of adhering to these guidelines.

Consistency and Follow-Through

Enforcing Boundaries Through Consistency

Consistency in the application of rules is essential for creating a predictable environment. It establishes an atmosphere where children understand the rules and the consequences for not following them. Consistency extends not only to the rules themselves but also to the enforcement of consequences outlined for non-compliance.

The Role of Follow-Through in Accountability

Addressing rule violations promptly and fairly is crucial. Rather than punitive measures alone, a constructive approach involving conversations about the reasons behind the violation and offering guidance on preventing similar incidents in the future is more effective. Maintaining accountability through constructive feedback reinforces the significance of adhering to the established rules.

Establishing clear and specific rules for social media usage within the family is fundamental for fostering a safe and responsible digital environment. These rules provide structure, promote responsible behavior, and contribute to a positive online experience. Effective communication, consistency in enforcement, and constructive handling of rule violations collectively empower families to navigate the digital landscape together, ensuring a healthier online experience for all members.

NEGOTIATING SCREEN TIME LIMITS

Process of Negotiation:

Negotiating screen time limits is a collaborative process that involves open communication and understanding between parents and children. It starts with creating a conducive environment for discussion, where everyone's views and concerns are heard and valued.

Initiating this negotiation involves:

Open Dialogue

Encouraging an open discussion where children can express their thoughts and concerns about screen usage without fear of judgment. This helps in establishing the groundwork for setting limits and objectives.

Involving Children

The involvement of children in decision-making is crucial. It not only helps them understand the reasons behind limitations but also gives them a sense of responsibility and ownership. Children who actively participate in setting boundaries are more likely to respect and abide by them.

Finding a Balance

Striking a balance between allowing social media use and maintaining healthy boundaries requires thoughtful strategies tailored to individual needs and developmental stages.

Strategies for achieving this balance include:

Prioritizing Activities

Emphasizing activities beyond screen time, such as physical exercise, family time, and hobbies, is essential. Balancing screen time with other activities promotes a healthier lifestyle.

Consistency and Flexibility

Maintaining consistent rules while being flexible enough to adapt to different situations, such as holidays or special events, ensures a more adaptable approach to screen time management.

Considering individual needs and developmental stages is crucial. This includes recognizing that younger children might need more guidance and stricter limits, while older children might require more autonomy with reasonable supervision.

Tips for Engaging Children:

Effectively engaging children in discussions about screen time involves fostering open communication and collaboration.

Effective engagement tips include:

Active Listening

Actively listening to children's perspectives without judgment encourages open and honest communication. Children are more likely to express their thoughts when they feel heard and understood.

Explaining Rationales

Clearly explaining the reasons behind screen time limits helps children understand the importance of balance and its positive impact on their overall well-being. This explanation encourages their cooperation in setting and adhering to limits.

Collaboration and Compromise

Encouraging collaboration between parents and children fosters a sense of joint responsibility in establishing mutually agreeable boundaries. This collaborative approach allows for negotiation and compromise, leading to boundaries that are acceptable to both parties.

Negotiating screen time limits involves fostering open dialogue, considering individual needs, and collaborating between parents and children. Engaging children in these discussions not only empowers them but also creates an environment for mutual understanding and compliance with established boundaries. The process emphasizes open communication, developmental considerations, and the active involvement of both parents and children in decision-making to achieve a harmonious balance in screen time usage within the family.

USING PARENTAL CONTROL TOOLS AND APPS

Parental control tools and apps serve as a crucial support system for parents navigating their children's online activities. These tools offer a range of functionalities designed to supervise and regulate social media usage, promoting a safer and more controlled digital environment.

Highlighting Available Tools

Overview of Parental Control Tools

Numerous parental control tools and apps cater to managing children's social media usage. Some prominent examples include Qustodio, Norton Family, Kaspersky Safe Kids, Family Link by Google, and Bark. These tools vary in features but share the common goal of assisting parents in overseeing their kids' online interactions.

Relevance in Promoting a Safe Environment

In the ever-expanding digital landscape, these tools are essential for parents to safeguard their children against cyber threats, inappropriate content exposure, cyberbullying, and online predators. By employing these tools, parents can actively engage in their children's online experiences, ensuring a secure and responsible digital presence.

Features and Benefits

Content Filtering

Parental control tools offer robust content filtering capabilities. This feature empowers parents to block or filter inappropriate websites, apps, or content categories based on their child's age and maturity level. It significantly minimizes exposure to harmful content.

Time Restrictions

The ability to set time limits on screen usage is another vital feature. Parents can regulate the amount of time children spend on social media or online activities, promoting a healthy balance between screen time and other activities.

Monitoring and Reporting

These tools provide real-time monitoring and comprehensive reports of children's online activities. Parents can track visited websites, social media interactions, messages, and search history. These insights enable informed discussions about responsible online behavior.

Remote Control and Location Tracking

Some parental control tools offer remote control functionalities, allowing parents to manage device access even when physically distant. Additionally, location tracking features aid in ensuring children's safety by allowing parents to monitor their whereabouts through GPS technology.

Benefits of Features

Collectively, these features contribute to fostering a safer and more balanced online experience for children. Content filtering protects them from harmful material, while time restrictions encourage healthy screen habits. Monitoring capabilities facilitate open communication between parents and children, promoting a safer digital environment.

Implementation and Utilization Tips

Open Communication

Initiate open and honest conversations with children about online safety and the purpose of using parental control tools. Encourage dialogue to establish trust and understanding.

Set Clear Rules and Expectations

Establish clear guidelines regarding screen time, permissible content, and online conduct. Explain the reasons behind these rules to garner cooperation from children.

Customize Settings According to Age

Adjust parental control settings based on each child's age, maturity, and individual needs. Regularly review and modify settings as children grow and exhibit responsible behavior.

Regularly Review Reports and Adjust Settings

Consistently monitor and review reports generated by these tools. Use this information to engage in discussions and modify settings if necessary to adapt to changing circumstances and evolving online behavior.

By leveraging these parental control tools and implementing them effectively, parents can actively participate in shaping a safer and more secure online environment for their children, allowing them to navigate the digital world responsibly and confidently.

4

BUILDING A STRONG CONNECTION

In today's digital age, where technology often takes center stage in our lives, building a strong connection with our children has become more important than ever. The digital world can sometimes hinder our ability to connect with our children on a deeper level, but it's essential that we prioritize and cultivate these relationships. This chapter will focus on techniques to reconnect with children and strengthen family relationships. We will begin by highlighting the importance of creating meaningful connections in the digital age and then explore strategies to achieve this.

The Importance of Meaningful Connections

In an era characterized by constant digital distractions, fostering meaningful connections with our children has never been more critical. Technology, while undoubtedly beneficial in many ways, can inadvertently lead to disconnection within families if not managed mindfully. As parents, it's essential that we recognize the significance of creating strong bonds with our children. These connections serve as the foundation for their emotional well-being, personal development, and overall happiness.

In today's fast-paced world, the following factors underscore the importance of building meaningful connections with our children:

Digital Overload

The prevalence of screens and digital devices often competes for our children's attention, potentially reducing the quality time spent together as a family.

Mental Health Challenges

The digital age has brought with it new challenges related to mental health, including increased feelings of isolation and anxiety. Building strong connections with our children can serve as a protective factor against these issues.

Emotional Support

Children need emotional support and guidance from their parents to navigate the complexities of life. Meaningful connections provide a safe space for children to express their thoughts, feelings, and concerns.

Positive Development

Strong family relationships contribute to the positive development of children. These relationships provide them with a sense of security, self-worth, and belonging.

Strategies for Building Strong Connections

Building a strong connection with your children is an ongoing process that requires effort, understanding, and patience. Here, we will explore several strategies that can help you reconnect with your children and strengthen family relationships:

Quality Time Over Quantity

While it's important to spend time with your children regularly, focus on the quality of the time spent together rather than just the quantity. Engage in activities that promote interaction and bonding, such as playing board games, cooking together, or going for a family hike. These shared experiences create lasting memories and deepen your connection.

Active Listening

Effective communication is at the heart of building strong connections. Practice active listening when your children speak, giving them your full attention. Avoid interrupting, and ask open-ended questions to encourage them to express themselves. Show empathy and understanding, validating their feelings and experiences.

Digital-Free Zones

Designate specific areas in your home as digital-free zones or times during which screens are put away. For example, the dining table can be a screen-free zone during family meals. These restrictions create opportunities for face-to-face interactions and meaningful conversations.

Set a Positive Example

Children learn by observing their parents. Be a role model for healthy screen time habits and interpersonal relationships. Demonstrate respect, kindness, and effective communication in your interactions with family members and others. Your behavior sets the tone for your children's behavior. **Share Interests**

Find common interests and hobbies that you can enjoy together. Whether it's reading, cooking, gardening, or playing a musical instrument, shared interests provide opportunities for bonding and collaboration.

Family Meetings

Hold regular family meetings where everyone has a chance to share their thoughts, feelings, and concerns. These meetings foster open communication and allow children to feel heard and valued within the family dynamic.

Be Present

When spending time with your children, be fully present in the moment. Put away distractions, including your phone, and focus on the activity or conversation at hand. This demonstrates your commitment to building a connection.

Support Individuality

Recognize and celebrate each child's unique personality, interests, and talents. Avoid making comparisons between siblings and allow each child to explore their individuality. This promotes a sense of self-worth and acceptance.

Teach Empathy

Empathy is a crucial component of meaningful connections. Teach your children to understand and consider the feelings of others. Encourage acts of kindness and empathy within the family and the broader community.

Create Family Traditions

Establishing family traditions, whether it's a weekly game night, an annual camping trip, or holiday rituals, creates a sense of belonging and continuity. These traditions provide opportunities for bonding and shared experiences.

Support Independence

As your children grow, encourage their independence and decision-making. Provide guidance and support while allowing them to explore their interests and learn from their experiences. This fosters a sense of autonomy and selfconfidence.

Offer Emotional Support

Let your children know that they can turn to you for emotional support and guidance. Create a safe and nonjudgmental space where they feel comfortable discussing their feelings and concerns.

Practice Gratitude

Encourage the practice of gratitude within the family. Expressing gratitude for one another and the positive aspects of family life strengthens the emotional connection and fosters a sense of appreciation.

Apologize and Forgive

In any relationship, misunderstandings and conflicts can arise. Teach your children the importance of apologizing when they are wrong and forgiving others when they make mistakes. These actions promote empathy, understanding, and reconciliation.

Be Patient

Building strong connections takes time, and there will be moments of frustration and challenges. Be patient and persistent in your efforts to strengthen your family relationships. The investment in these connections is immeasurable.

In our increasingly digital world, the importance of creating meaningful connections with our children cannot be overstated. These connections serve as the cornerstone of their emotional well-being and personal development. By implementing these strategies, you can not only reconnect with your children but also nurture strong, loving, and lasting family relationships that will endure through the challenges of the digital age.

CREATING TECH-FREE ZONES AND QUALITY BONDING TIME

In our digital age, where screens and devices often dominate our lives, it's crucial to establish tech-free zones and prioritize quality bonding time within the family. These practices serve as a counterbalance to the pervasive presence of technology, promoting face-to-face interaction and strengthening familial connections. In this section, we will delve into the importance of designated tech-free zones, practical strategies for setting boundaries, and the pivotal role of parental example in shaping children's attitudes toward technology usage.

Importance of Designated Tech-Free Zones

Promoting Face-to-Face Interaction

Designating specific areas or times in the home as techfree zones is instrumental in fostering face-to-face interaction among family members. In these zones, screens are put aside, creating opportunities for genuine conversations, active listening, and non-digital connections.

Strengthening Familial Connections

Tech-free zones provide a space where family members can connect on a deeper level. They encourage meaningful conversations, laughter, and shared experiences that contribute to stronger bonds and emotional connections within the family unit.

Enhancing Well-Being

Stepping away from screens in designated tech-free zones allows individuals, especially children, to disconnect from the constant stimulation of digital devices. This respite can lead to reduced stress, improved mental well-being, and better sleep quality.

Fostering Discipline and Self-Control

Tech-free zones teach children the importance of setting boundaries and practicing self-control when it comes to technology use. These experiences can carry over into other aspects of their digital lives.

Strategies for Setting Boundaries

Define Tech-Free Zones

Identify specific areas in your home where screens are not allowed. Common examples include the dining room during meals, bedrooms before bedtime, and family gathering spaces.

Allocate specific times as tech-free, such as designated hours after school or during family activities.

Establish Clear Rules

Create clear and age-appropriate rules regarding technology use in tech-free zones. Ensure that every family member understands these rules and the consequences for violating them.

Use positive reinforcement to reward compliance with the rules. Praise and encourage children when they adhere to the boundaries.

Communicate Expectations

Openly communicate the reasons behind tech-free zones and boundaries. Explain to your children the benefits of face-toface interaction, quality bonding time, and the importance of managing screen time responsibly.

Encourage your children to express their thoughts and concerns about these rules. Involving them in the discussion can foster a sense of ownership and understanding.

Create Alternatives

Provide alternative activities for family members during tech-free times. This could include playing board games, engaging in outdoor activities, reading together, or pursuing shared hobbies.

Ensure that these alternatives are enjoyable and appealing, making it more likely for family members to willingly participate.

Use Technology Tools

Leverage technology itself to help set boundaries. Many smartphones and devices come equipped with parental control features that allow you to restrict access to specific apps or websites during certain times.

Explore parental control software and apps that can help monitor and manage screen time for children.

Be Consistent

Consistency is key in enforcing boundaries. Stick to the established rules and boundaries consistently to create a sense of predictability and routine within the family.

If necessary, hold family meetings to remind everyone of the rules and discuss any adjustments or concerns.

Leading by Example

Prioritize Device-Free Time

Parents should actively prioritize and demonstrate the importance of device-free time. This includes setting aside screens during family meals, activities, and quality bonding moments.

When children observe their parents valuing face-to-face interactions over screens, they are more likely to emulate these behaviors.

Engage in Shared Activities

Participate in shared activities that do not involve screens. Engaging in these activities as a family sets a powerful example for children, emphasizing the value of quality bonding time.

Whether it's going for a hike, playing board games, or cooking together, these experiences create lasting memories and connections.

Communicate Openly

Maintain open communication with your children about your own relationship with technology. Share your own challenges and successes in managing screen time.

Encourage your children to ask questions and express their concerns about your technology use. This dialogue can lead to a deeper understanding of the role of technology in daily life.

Set Screen Time Limits for Everyone

Apply screen time limits and boundaries to every family member, including parents. This demonstrates a sense of fairness and equality within the family dynamic.

When parents adhere to the same boundaries they set for their children, it reinforces the idea that these rules apply to everyone.

Be Mindful of Screen Use in Social Settings

Model appropriate screen use in social settings. When attending family gatherings, outings, or events, focus on engaging with others rather than constantly checking your devices.

Demonstrate the importance of being present and attentive during social interactions.

Embrace Digital Detoxes

Lead by example in embracing digital detoxes. Encourage the entire family to participate in periods of screenfree time together.

Use these detoxes as an opportunity to connect, engage in activities, and enjoy each other's company without the distractions of screens.

creating tech-free zones, setting boundaries, and leading by example are essential strategies for fostering meaningful connections within the family. In the digital age, where screens often dominate our lives, it's crucial to carve out time and spaces for genuine face-to-face interactions and quality bonding moments. By implementing these strategies and prioritizing relationships over screens, parents can set a positive example and create a nurturing environment where strong family connections can thrive.

ACTIVE LISTENING AND OPEN COMMUNICATION

Significance of Active Listening

Effective communication is the cornerstone of building strong connections with children. In this digital age, where distractions abound, active listening plays a pivotal role in creating meaningful interactions with our children. It's not merely hearing words but fully engaging in the process of understanding and empathizing with what our children are expressing. Let's explore further the importance of active listening in strengthening parent-child relationships.

Building Strong Connections

Active listening is the bridge that connects parents and children on an emotional level. When we actively listen to our children, we convey that their thoughts, feelings, and opinions are valued and respected. This sense of value and respect is foundational for building strong connections. Children thrive in an environment where they feel heard and understood.

Understanding and Empathy

Active listening goes beyond the surface of words. It delves into the nuances of emotions and experiences that our children are trying to convey. It allows us to walk in their shoes momentarily, gaining profound insights into their perspectives, emotions, and needs. This understanding is the bedrock of empathy, which is essential for effective parenting.

Strengthening Parent-Child Relationships

At its core, active listening is about creating a space where our children feel safe to express themselves. When they sense that their voices matter and that they can share their thoughts and feelings without judgment or ridicule, it strengthens the parent-child relationship. Such an environment encourages trust, openness, and a genuine connection that extends beyond the surface of everyday conversations.

Practical Techniques for Parents

Understanding the significance of active listening is one thing; applying it in our daily interactions with our children is another. Let's delve into practical techniques that parents can adopt to enhance their active listening skills.

Maintain Eye Contact

Maintaining eye contact during a conversation may seem like a small gesture, but it carries significant weight. It signals to your child that you are fully present and engaged in the interaction. When you look into their eyes, they feel seen, heard, and respected.

Paraphrasing

After your child has shared their thoughts or feelings, take a moment to paraphrase what they've said. This involves rephrasing their words in your own to confirm your understanding. For example, you can say, "So, if I understand correctly, you're feeling..." Paraphrasing not only validates their perspective but also ensures that you've accurately grasped their message.

Ask Open-Ended Questions

Encourage your child to share more by asking openended questions. These are questions that cannot be answered with a simple "yes" or "no." Open-ended questions invite your child to elaborate and provide more detailed responses. For instance, instead of asking, "Did you have a good day at school?" you can inquire, "What was the most interesting thing that happened at school today?"

Reflect Feelings

Pay close attention to your child's emotional cues during the conversation. When you detect a particular emotion, reflect it back to them. For example, you can say, "It sounds like you felt really happy when that happened," or "I can see that you were upset by that." Reflecting their feelings not only shows that you're attuned to their emotions but also validates their right to feel the way they do.

Minimize Distractions

In today's digital age, distractions are abundant. To engage in active listening effectively, create a distraction-free environment. Put away your phone, turn off the TV, and find a quiet space where you can focus solely on the conversation. Eliminating distractions sends a clear message that your child's words are a priority.

Avoid Interrupting

Patience is a virtue in active listening. Resist the urge to interrupt when your child is speaking. Let them finish expressing themselves before responding. Interrupting can disrupt the flow of their thoughts and discourage open communication.

Be Patient

Give your child the time they need to gather their thoughts and express themselves. Don't rush the conversation or push for immediate answers. Patience allows your child to feel more comfortable and less pressured during discussions.

These practical techniques can be incorporated into everyday interactions with your child, enhancing your ability to actively listen and, in turn, strengthening your connection with them.

Creating a Safe and Non-Judgmental Environment

Active listening is most effective when it takes place within a safe and non-judgmental environment. Let's delve into the importance of fostering such an atmosphere for children to express their thoughts and feelings openly.

Embrace Empathy

Empathy is the cornerstone of creating a safe space for your child to communicate. It involves understanding and sharing in your child's feelings, even if those feelings differ from your own. When you approach your child's emotions with empathy, it communicates that you care about their well-being and that their feelings are valid.

Be Non-Judgmental

A non-judgmental stance is essential in fostering open communication. Children need to feel that they can express themselves without fear of criticism or condemnation. Avoid making hasty judgments or reacting negatively to their words. Instead, listen with an open mind, seeking to understand their perspective.

Encourage Openness

From an early age, encourage your child to express themselves openly. Let them know that their thoughts and feelings are not just welcome but encouraged. Create an environment where they feel safe sharing anything on their mind, whether it's their hopes, fears, or concerns. This open-door policy promotes trust and strengthens the parent-child relationship.

Respect Privacy

Respect your child's need for privacy and personal space. While open communication is encouraged, avoid prying or invasive questions. Recognize that some matters may be private, and your child should be free to share at their own pace. Respecting their boundaries demonstrates that you trust and respect them as individuals.

Be Supportive

Support is a crucial component of a safe environment. Express your support and encouragement, especially when your child shares difficult or challenging experiences. Reassure them that you are there to help and guide them through life's ups and downs. Being supportive fosters a sense of security and reassurance.

Use Positive Reinforcement

Positive reinforcement plays a role in creating a culture of open communication within the family. Acknowledge and appreciate your child's efforts in communicating openly. Praise their willingness to share their thoughts and feelings. Positive reinforcement reinforces the importance of open communication and encourages its continuation.

Practice Active Listening as a Family

Make active listening a family practice. Encourage all family members, including siblings, to engage in active listening when someone is speaking. Create a culture of respect and understanding within the family where everyone's voice is heard and valued. This not only strengthens parent-child relationships but also enhances sibling relationships and the overall family dynamic.

Active listening, practical techniques for parents, and a safe and non-judgmental environment are crucial components of effective communication within the family. When parents actively listen to their children, they create a bond built on trust, empathy, and open communication. By fostering a safe and welcoming atmosphere, parents empower their children to express themselves freely, leading to deeper connections and stronger relationships within the family.

ENGAGING IN SHARED ACTIVITIES AND HOBBIES

Benefits of Shared Activities

Engaging in shared activities and hobbies as a family is a powerful way to strengthen family relationships and create lasting bonds. These activities offer numerous benefits that go beyond the immediate enjoyment of the activity itself. Let's explore the advantages of sharing activities and how they contribute to a sense of connection and mutual enjoyment within the family.

Quality Time Together

Shared activities provide an opportunity for families to spend quality time together. In today's fast-paced world, where everyone has busy schedules and digital distractions can dominate, carving out time for shared activities allows families to reconnect.

Strengthening Bonds

Participating in activities as a family strengthens the emotional bonds between family members. These shared experiences create memories that are cherished for years to come and foster a sense of togetherness.

Enhanced Communication

Engaging in shared activities encourages communication within the family. During these activities, family members talk, share ideas, and work together towards a common goal. This enhances overall communication skills and promotes open dialogue.

Building Trust

Collaborating on activities fosters trust and cooperation among family members. It teaches children that their family members are reliable and supportive, which can positively impact their overall sense of security.

Developing Life Skills

Many shared activities involve problem-solving, teamwork, and decision-making, which are essential life skills. Engaging in these activities as a family provides a practical and fun way to develop these skills.

Creating Traditions

Shared activities can become family traditions, whether it's a weekly game night, an annual camping trip, or holiday rituals. These traditions provide a sense of continuity and create a strong family identity.

Mutual Enjoyment

Shared activities often lead to mutual enjoyment. When family members participate in something they all find fun or interesting, it reinforces positive feelings and shared interests.

Types of Activities

The versatility of shared activities allows families to choose from a wide range of options, catering to different interests, ages, and abilities. Here are some types of activities that families can enjoy together:

Cooking and Baking

Preparing meals together can be a delightful and educational activity. Family members can take turns selecting recipes, shopping for ingredients, and cooking or baking as a team. It's an opportunity to bond while learning about nutrition and culinary skills.

Gardening

Gardening provides a hands-on way to connect with nature and each other. Families can plant flowers, vegetables, or herbs together, nurturing a shared project that yields both beauty and fresh produce.

Sports and Outdoor Activities

Participating in sports or outdoor activities like hiking, biking, or playing soccer encourages physical fitness and teamwork. These activities promote a healthy lifestyle while fostering cooperation and friendly competition.

Arts and Crafts

Artistic pursuits such as painting, drawing, pottery, or crafting offer a creative outlet for family members. Everyone can express themselves and work on artistic projects together, resulting in unique and meaningful creations.

Board Games and Puzzles

Board games and puzzles are excellent for family game nights. They stimulate critical thinking, problem-solving, and healthy competition. These activities can be adjusted to suit different age levels.

Reading Together

Reading books as a family allows for shared literary experiences and discussions. Choose age-appropriate books and take turns reading aloud, or discuss the stories and themes as you go along.

Home Improvement Projects

Working on home improvement projects, such as painting a room, building furniture, or renovating spaces, not only enhances your living environment but also provides a sense of accomplishment and teamwork.

Volunteering

Participating in volunteer activities as a family can be deeply rewarding. It instills a sense of social responsibility and empathy in children while allowing the family to bond over shared values.

Music and Dance

Exploring music and dance as a family can be a joyful experience. Singing, playing musical instruments, or simply dancing to your favorite tunes in the living room can create lasting memories.

Outdoor Adventures

Embarking on outdoor adventures like camping, fishing, or boating allows families to connect with nature and disconnect from digital distractions. These experiences often lead to shared stories and laughter around the campfire.

Identifying Children's Interests

To select the most suitable shared activities, it's essential for parents to identify their children's interests and passions.

Here are some practical suggestions on how to do this:

Observe and Listen

Pay close attention to your children's interests by observing what they naturally gravitate toward and listening to their conversations. Children often drop hints about their passions through their words and actions.

Ask Open-Ended Questions

Engage your children in conversations that encourage them to express their interests and preferences. Ask open-ended questions like, "What do you enjoy doing in your free time?" or

"What topics at school fascinate you the most?"

Explore a Variety of Activities

Expose your children to a variety of activities and hobbies. Enroll them in classes or workshops that cover different areas of interest, from sports to arts and sciences. This allows them to discover what resonates with them.

Encourage Curiosity

Foster a sense of curiosity in your children by supporting their exploration of different subjects and hobbies. Provide access to books, documentaries, museums, and experiences that can spark their interests.

Be Supportive, Not Pushy

While it's essential to encourage your children to explore their passions, avoid pressuring them into specific activities. Let their interests develop naturally, and support them without imposing your own expectations.

Create Opportunities for Exploration

Set aside time and resources for your children to explore their interests. Whether it's signing them up for a dance class, visiting a science museum, or enrolling them in a sports league, create opportunities for them to delve deeper into their chosen activities.

Join Them in Their Interests

Once you've identified your children's interests, consider joining them in their pursuits. Whether you share the same passion or not, your active participation shows that you value their interests and are willing to engage in shared activities that bring you closer as a family.

Engaging in shared activities and hobbies as a family offers a wealth of benefits, from strengthening bonds to creating lasting memories. The versatility of these activities allows families to tailor their choices to suit their interests and preferences. By actively listening to their children, parents can identify their passions and create opportunities for connection and shared enjoyment. Whether it's cooking together, embarking on outdoor adventures, or nurturing artistic talents, shared activities foster a sense of togetherness that contributes to a harmonious and connected family life.

5
RECOGNIZING AND ADDRESSING ADDICTION

RECOGNIZING AND ADDRESSING SOCIAL MEDIA ADDICTION

In today's digital age, social media has become an integral part of our lives, especially for younger generations. It offers numerous benefits, such as connecting with friends and family, staying updated on current events, and even networking for personal and professional growth. However, there is a growing concern about the negative consequences of excessive social media use, which has led to the emergence of social media addiction. In this chapter, we will focus on educating parents about the signs of social media addiction and providing strategies for addressing it. We will also emphasize the importance of early recognition and intervention to mitigate the impact of excessive social media use on individuals and their families.

Understanding Social Media Addiction

Social media addiction, also known as social media dependency or problematic social media use, refers to a condition where individuals develop a compulsive and unhealthy relationship with social media platforms. They may find it challenging to control the amount of time they spend on social media, leading to detrimental effects on various aspects of their lives, including their physical and mental health, academic or professional performance, and relationships.

Recognizing the Signs

Recognizing the signs of social media addiction is the first step in addressing this issue effectively. Parents play a crucial role in identifying these signs in their children. Here are some common signs to look out for:

Excessive Time Spent Online

One of the most apparent signs is spending an excessive amount of time on social media platforms. This includes late nights spent scrolling through feeds and checking notifications during important activities.

Neglecting Responsibilities

Social media addiction can lead to neglecting essential responsibilities such as schoolwork, household chores, or workrelated tasks. A decline in academic or professional performance may be indicative of this.

Withdrawal Symptoms

When individuals are unable to access their social media accounts, they may experience symptoms similar to withdrawal, such as irritability, anxiety, or restlessness.

Neglecting Real-Life Relationships

Excessive social media use often results in neglecting face-to-face relationships with friends and family. Individuals may prefer virtual interactions over real-life ones.

Deteriorating Mental Health

Social media addiction can contribute to deteriorating mental health, including symptoms of depression, anxiety, and low self-esteem. Constant comparison with others on social media can lead to negative self-perception.

Preoccupation with Likes and Followers

An obsession with gaining likes, followers, and comments on social media posts can be a telltale sign of addiction. The validation from online interactions becomes more critical than real-life connections.

Privacy Invasion

Sharing excessive personal information and photos online, even when it compromises one's privacy or safety, can be a sign of social media addiction.

Inability to Disconnect

Individuals addicted to social media find it challenging to disconnect voluntarily. They may check their phones or log in to social media accounts even in situations where it's inappropriate or unsafe, such as while driving.

The Importance of Early Recognition and Intervention

Early recognition and intervention are crucial when dealing with social media addiction. The impact of excessive social media use on an individual's life can escalate rapidly, affecting their physical and mental health, academic or professional prospects, and relationships with others. Here's why early intervention is essential:

Preventing Long-term Consequences

The longer social media addiction goes untreated, the more profound its impact becomes. Early intervention can prevent long-term consequences and minimize the harm caused by excessive use.

Preserving Relationships

Recognizing addiction early allows for the preservation of real-life relationships that may have suffered due to neglect. This can prevent long-lasting damage to family bonds and friendships.

Enhancing Mental Health

Addressing social media addiction at an early stage can help improve an individual's mental health. Reducing the negative emotions associated with excessive use, such as anxiety and depression, can have a significant positive impact on wellbeing.

Improving Academic and Professional Success

Students and professionals alike may experience a decline in their performance due to social media addiction. Early intervention can help them regain focus and improve their academic or career prospects.

Strategies for Addressing Social Media Addiction

Once parents recognize the signs of social media addiction in their children, it's essential to have effective strategies for addressing the issue. Here are some strategies to consider:

Open Communication

Start by having an open and non-judgmental conversation with your child. Express your concerns and listen to their perspective. Avoid blaming or shaming them, as this can lead to defensiveness.

Set Healthy Boundaries

Work together to establish clear boundaries for social media use. This includes defining specific time limits and designated "tech-free" zones, such as during meals or family activities.

Lead by Example

Children often learn by observing their parents' behavior. Set a positive example by managing your own social media use and demonstrating a healthy balance between online and offline activities.

Encourage Offline Activities

Encourage your child to participate in offline activities they enjoy, such as sports, hobbies, or spending time with friends in person. These activities can help fill the void left by reduced social media use.

Seek Professional Help

If the addiction is severe and causing significant harm, consider seeking professional help. Therapists and counselors who specialize in addiction can provide valuable guidance and support.

Monitor Online Friends and Content

Pay attention to your child's online connections and the content they consume. Ensure they are not engaging with harmful or inappropriate content or interacting with strangers.

Install Parental Control Software

Consider using parental control software to monitor and limit your child's online activities. These tools can help enforce time limits and provide insights into their online behavior.

Encourage Self-reflection

Help your child develop self-awareness about their social media use. Encourage them to reflect on how it makes them feel and whether it is adding value to their lives.

Build Offline Connections

Support your child in building and maintaining offline friendships. Arrange playdates or outings with friends to reinforce the importance of real-life relationships.

Celebrate Progress:

Acknowledge and celebrate your child's efforts to reduce their social media use and make positive changes in their life. Positive reinforcement can motivate continued improvement.

In a world dominated by social media, recognizing and addressing addiction is paramount, especially when it comes to our children.

Social media addiction can have severe consequences on their well-being, relationships, and future prospects. This chapter has highlighted the importance of early recognition and intervention and provided strategies for parents to address social media addiction in their children.

By staying vigilant, maintaining open communication, and fostering a healthy balance between online and offline activities, parents can help their children develop a healthier relationship with social media. The goal is not to eliminate social media use entirely but to ensure that it enriches their lives rather than becoming a source of addiction and harm. With the right approach, parents can play a crucial role in guiding their children towards a balanced and fulfilling digital life.

BEHAVIORAL INDICATORS OF ADDICTION

Recognition of Addictive Behaviors

The ubiquitous nature of social media has transformed the way we connect, communicate, and consume information. While social media platforms offer many benefits, they also carry the potential for addiction, which can significantly impact an individual's life. In this section, we will discuss how excessive social media use can lead to addictive behaviors and explore common behavioral indicators that can help recognize social media addiction.

Excessive Social Media Use as an Addiction

Addiction is a complex condition characterized by the compulsive engagement in rewarding stimuli despite adverse consequences. When it comes to social media, the constant availability of social validation, novel content, and the fear of missing out (FOMO) can create a perfect storm for addictive behaviors.

Here's how excessive social media use can lead to addiction:

Instant Gratification

Social media platforms are designed to provide instant gratification. Likes, comments, and shares trigger the release of dopamine in the brain, the "feel-good" neurotransmitter. Over time, individuals may seek this dopamine rush by compulsively checking their social media accounts, much like a person addicted to drugs or alcohol seeks their substance of choice.

FOMO

The fear of missing out is a powerful motivator. When individuals see their friends and peers posting exciting and engaging content on social media, they may feel compelled to keep up. This fear of missing out can drive excessive use, even when it interferes with other aspects of life.

Escapism

Social media provides an easy escape from real-life stressors and challenges. People may turn to their online personas to avoid dealing with problems or negative emotions, further reinforcing their dependence on these platforms.

Social Comparison

Constantly comparing one's life to the seemingly perfect lives of others on social media can lead to feelings of inadequacy and a need to keep up. This can fuel addictive behaviors as individuals strive to present an idealized version of themselves online.

Reinforcement Loop

The algorithms used by social media platforms are designed to keep users engaged for as long as possible. They employ machine learning to understand user preferences and show content tailored to those preferences. This reinforcement loop can make it challenging for individuals to disengage from their social media accounts.

Now that we've explored how excessive social media use can lead to addictive behaviors let's delve into some of the common behavioral indicators that can help recognize social media addiction:

Withdrawal Symptoms

Withdrawal symptoms are a hallmark of addiction. In the context of social media, withdrawal symptoms may manifest as:

Irritability and Restlessness

Individuals addicted to social media may become irritable and restless when they are unable to access their accounts. This can be especially noticeable during periods without internet connectivity or when they are trying to cut down on their usage.

Anxiety

The fear of missing out or the anticipation of social media notifications can lead to anxiety when users are away from their screens. The constant need to check for updates can become overwhelming.

Depression

Social media withdrawal can also trigger feelings of sadness or depression. Individuals may feel isolated or excluded when they are not connected to their online social circles.

Preoccupation

Preoccupation with social media is a key behavioral indicator of addiction. This preoccupation may manifest in various ways:

Constant Checking

Individuals addicted to social media may feel compelled to check their accounts repeatedly, even in inappropriate or unsafe situations. This behavior can disrupt daily activities and responsibilities.

Obsessive Posting

Addiction can drive individuals to obsessively post updates, photos, or status messages on social media platforms, seeking validation and engagement from their online peers.

Excessive Time Online

Spending an inordinate amount of time on social media, often at the expense of other activities, is a clear sign of preoccupation. This can interfere with work, studies, and faceto-face relationships.

Neglect of Responsibilities

One of the most damaging consequences of social media addiction is the neglect of responsibilities, which can include:

Academic or Professional Decline

Addiction can lead to a decline in academic or professional performance as individuals prioritize social media over their studies or job responsibilities.

Household Chores

Neglecting household chores or responsibilities is common among those addicted to social media. This can strain relationships within the family and impact daily life.

Health and Self-care

Addiction may also result in neglecting one's physical and mental health, as individuals spend excessive amounts of time online at the expense of exercise, sleep, or self-care routines.

Negative Consequences

Addiction often leads to negative consequences, and social media addiction is no exception:

Strained Relationships

Excessive social media use can strain real-life relationships as individuals prioritize online interactions over face-to-face connections with friends and family.

Mental Health Issues

Social media addiction can contribute to mental health issues such as depression, anxiety, and low self-esteem. Constant comparison with others can lead to negative selfperception.

Privacy Concerns

Addiction may lead individuals to overshare personal information and compromise their privacy on social media platforms, which can have long-term consequences.

Financial Impact

In some cases, social media addiction can result in financial consequences when individuals spend money on virtual items or experiences within social media platforms.

Recognizing these behavioral indicators is crucial for identifying social media addiction and taking steps to address it effectively. In the next section, we will explore strategies for addressing social media addiction and promoting a healthier relationship with these platforms.

SEEKING PROFESSIONAL HELP AND SUPPORT

Importance of Professional Intervention

Addressing social media addiction often requires professional assistance, as it can be a challenging and complex issue to overcome. While recognizing the signs and behavioral indicators of addiction is crucial, it's equally important to understand the significance of seeking professional help in the recovery process. In this section, we will emphasize the importance of professional intervention and discuss the potential benefits of involving therapists, counselors, or support groups when dealing with social media addiction.

Recognition of the Need for Professional Help

Social media addiction can be deeply ingrained in an individual's life, affecting their mental health, relationships, and overall well-being. Recognizing the need for professional intervention is a vital step in addressing this issue effectively.

Here are some reasons why professional help is essential:

Expertise and Specialization

Trained professionals, such as therapists and counselors, have the expertise and specialization required to understand the complexities of addiction. They can assess the severity of the addiction and tailor treatment plans accordingly.

Objective Assessment

Professionals offer an objective perspective on the situation, which can be especially valuable when dealing with a loved one's addiction. They can provide an unbiased assessment of the problem and recommend appropriate interventions.

Evidence-Based Approaches

Therapists and counselors use evidence-based approaches and therapeutic techniques that have proven to be effective in treating addiction. These methods are grounded in research and clinical experience.

Support and Guidance

Addiction recovery can be emotionally challenging, and individuals often need emotional support and guidance. Professionals can provide a safe and supportive environment for individuals and their families to navigate the recovery process.

Potential Benefits of Involving Professionals

When seeking help for social media addiction, involving therapists, counselors, or support groups can yield several significant benefits:

Customized Treatment Plans

Professionals can assess the unique needs and challenges of individuals struggling with social media addiction and create customized treatment plans. These plans may include strategies to address underlying issues, such as anxiety or depression.

Behavioral Modification

Therapists can help individuals identify and modify the specific behaviors that contribute to addiction. This may involve teaching coping skills and alternative ways to manage stress or negative emotions.

Family Support

Addiction affects not only the individual but also their family members. Professionals can facilitate family therapy sessions to improve communication, set boundaries, and provide support to everyone involved.

Peer Support

Support groups, either in-person or online, offer individuals the opportunity to connect with others who are experiencing similar challenges. Sharing experiences and insights in a group setting can be empowering and reduce feelings of isolation.

Relapse Prevention

Professionals can help individuals develop relapse prevention strategies to maintain their recovery over the long term. These strategies may involve identifying triggers and learning healthy ways to cope with them.

Guidance on Seeking Appropriate Support

Parents who recognize that their child is struggling with social media addiction may wonder how to seek the appropriate professional support. Here's practical guidance on how to identify and access the right assistance for their child:

Start with Communication

Begin by discussing your concerns with your child. Express your willingness to support them in seeking help. Encourage open and honest communication about their addiction.

Consult with a Pediatrician

If you are uncertain about the severity of the addiction or its impact on your child's health, consider consulting with a pediatrician. They can provide guidance and may refer you to mental health professionals if necessary.

Research Therapists and Counselors

Look for therapists or counselors who specialize in addiction, preferably those with experience in treating social media addiction or internet-related disorders. Online directories, recommendations from trusted sources, and referrals from medical professionals can help in this search.

Check Credentials

Ensure that the professionals you consider are licensed and accredited in their respective fields. You can verify their credentials through state licensing boards or professional organizations.

Interview Potential Professionals

Schedule initial consultations or interviews with potential therapists or counselors. Use these meetings to ask questions about their approach to treatment, experience with social media addiction, and how they involve family members in the recovery process.

Consider Support Groups

Explore local or online support groups dedicated to addiction recovery. These groups can provide valuable peer support and insights. Organizations like SMART Recovery and 12-Step programs may have specific groups for internet or social media addiction.

Insurance Coverage

Check with your health insurance provider to understand the coverage for mental health services. This can help you manage the cost of professional assistance.

Involvement of Trained Professionals

Trained professionals play a crucial role in guiding both parents and children through the recovery process from social media addiction. Here are some insights into their role:

Assessment and Diagnosis

Professionals conduct thorough assessments to diagnose the severity of the addiction and any underlying mental health issues. This assessment serves as the foundation for developing an effective treatment plan.

Individual Therapy

Individual therapy sessions provide a safe and confidential space for individuals to explore the factors contributing to their addiction. Therapists use various therapeutic techniques to help clients understand their behaviors and work towards change.

Family Therapy

Family therapy sessions involve the entire family in the recovery process. This can help improve communication, address conflicts, and provide support to both the individual with addiction and their loved ones.

Crisis Intervention

In some cases, addiction may lead to crisis situations. Trained professionals can provide crisis intervention and ensure the safety of the individual. They can also coordinate with emergency services if necessary.

Monitoring and Progress Tracking

Professionals monitor the progress of individuals in recovery, adjusting treatment plans as needed. They help individuals set goals and track their achievements, providing motivation and encouragement.

Relapse Prevention

Professionals work with individuals to develop relapse prevention strategies. These strategies help individuals recognize and cope with triggers and stressors that may lead to a relapse.

Seeking professional help and support is a critical component of addressing social media addiction. Trained professionals bring expertise, objectivity, and evidence-based approaches to the recovery process. Parents can play an essential role in guiding their children towards appropriate professional assistance, ensuring that they receive the specialized care needed to overcome social media addiction and regain control of their lives.

Setting Clear Boundaries

Setting clear boundaries is crucial for establishing a healthier relationship with technology, especially when addressing social media addiction. These boundaries provide structure and guidance, helping individuals regain control over their screen time. Let's discuss the importance of setting clear boundaries and explore practical techniques for defining and enforcing them regarding social media use.

Importance of Setting Clear Boundaries

Preventing Overuse

Boundaries help individuals avoid excessive use of social media by setting limits on the time spent online. This prevents addiction from escalating.

Balancing Screen Time

Clear boundaries promote a healthy balance between screen time and offline activities. This ensures that social media does not dominate an individual's life.

Prioritizing Responsibilities

Boundaries encourage individuals to prioritize their responsibilities, such as schoolwork, chores, and personal wellbeing, over social media use.

Improving Sleep

Establishing boundaries around bedtime prevents latenight scrolling, which can negatively impact sleep quality and overall health.

Practical Techniques for Defining and Enforcing Boundaries

Set Specific Time Limits

Determine the maximum amount of time individuals are allowed to spend on social media each day. Use smartphone features or third-party apps to set timers or reminders.

Designate Tech-Free Zones

Designate certain areas in your home, such as the dining room or bedrooms, as tech-free zones. This encourages face-toface interactions and prevents mindless scrolling.

Establish Screen-Free Times

Define specific times of day when social media is offlimits, such as during meals, study or work hours, and before bedtime.

Use Parental Control Software

If you're a parent concerned about your child's social media use, consider using parental control software to enforce time limits and restrict access to certain apps or websites.

Create a Family Media Plan

Collaboratively develop a family media plan that outlines guidelines and expectations for screen time. Involve all family members in the discussion to ensure a sense of ownership.

Model Healthy Behavior

Lead by example by demonstrating healthy screen time habits. When children see their parents setting and adhering to boundaries, they are more likely to do the same.

Regularly Review and Adjust

Periodically review and adjust the established boundaries to ensure they remain effective and relevant. As circumstances change, so too should the boundaries.

Encouraging Alternative Activities

Encouraging children to engage in alternative activities beyond social media is essential for reducing dependence on screen time. Diversifying interests helps individuals find fulfillment and enjoyment in activities that do not involve technology. Here are strategies for promoting alternative activities:

Identify Interests and Passions

Encourage your child to explore their interests and passions, whether it's a sport, art, music, or a hobby. Engaging in activities they are passionate about can naturally reduce the time spent on social media.

Set Goals

Help your child set achievable goals related to their interests. These goals provide motivation and a sense of accomplishment, which can be more rewarding than social media interactions.

Plan Offline Outings

Organize family outings or activities that do not involve screens. This could include hiking, picnics, board games, or volunteering in the community.

Limit Screen Time Gradually

If your child's screen time is currently excessive, consider reducing it gradually. This gives them time to adapt to the change and discover alternative activities.

Encourage Reading

Reading books, magazines, or even online articles unrelated to social media can be a fulfilling alternative. Foster a love for reading and critical thinking.

Sports and Physical Activities

Encourage participation in sports or physical activities that promote physical fitness and social interaction. Team sports, martial arts, and yoga are excellent options.

Creative Outlets

Support creative outlets such as writing, drawing, painting, or playing a musical instrument. Creative activities provide a sense of accomplishment and self-expression.

Promoting Digital Detoxes

Digital detoxes are intentional breaks from screens and technology, allowing individuals to reset their relationship with social media and other digital platforms. They play a crucial role in reducing dependence on social media and promoting a healthier balance in technology usage. Here's an examination of the concept of digital detoxes and practical tips on implementing them:

The Role of Digital Detoxes

Breaking Habitual Behaviors

Digital detoxes interrupt the cycle of compulsive social media use, allowing individuals to regain control over their screen time.

Restoring Mental Well-being

Detoxes provide an opportunity to focus on mental and emotional well-being, reducing stress and anxiety associated with constant digital connectivity.

Enhancing Productivity

Taking a break from social media can boost productivity by eliminating distractions and improving concentration.

Practical Tips for Implementing Digital Detoxes

Plan in Advance

Schedule digital detox periods in advance, ideally during weekends or holidays when work or school commitments are minimal.

Communicate the Detox

Inform friends, family, and social media contacts about your detox plans. This reduces the pressure to respond to notifications.

Set a Duration

Determine the duration of your detox, whether it's a day, a week-end, or an entire week. Start with a manageable timeframe and gradually increase it.

Find Offline Activities

Plan alternative activities to fill your time during the detox, such as spending time outdoors, pursuing hobbies, or engaging in face-to-face social interactions.

Use Apps for Assistance

There are apps designed to help individuals track and limit their screen time. Consider using such apps to enforce your detox.

Create a Support System

Involve family members or friends in your detox journey. Having a support system can make it easier to stay committed.

Reflect and Journal

Use the detox period to reflect on your relationship with social media and technology. Journaling your thoughts and feelings can provide valuable insights.

Fostering Open Communication

Fostering open communication between parents and children is paramount when addressing social media addiction. A supportive and non-judgmental environment encourages individuals to share their struggles and seek help. Here are communication strategies that create such an environment:

Active Listening

Practice active listening when your child talks about their social media use or addiction. Show empathy and understanding without immediately offering solutions or criticism.

Express Concerns

Share your concerns about your child's well-being and the impact of excessive social media use on their life. Be specific and provide examples of observed behaviors.

Avoid Blame and Judgment

Avoid blaming or shaming your child for their addiction. Instead, focus on the addiction as a challenge you can overcome together.

Offer Support

Let your child know that you are there to support them in their journey to reduce social media dependence. Offer assistance in finding professional help if needed.

Be Patient

Recognize that overcoming addiction takes time and effort. Be patient with your child's progress and setbacks, offering encouragement along the way.

Set Boundaries on Communication

Establish boundaries regarding communication about social media. Encourage open discussions but ensure that they do not become confrontational or invasive.

Collaborative Problem-Solving

Involve your child in problem-solving. Collaboratively explore solutions to reduce social media addiction, allowing them to have a say in their recovery.

Implementing strategies for reducing dependence on social media involves setting clear boundaries, encouraging alternative activities, promoting digital detoxes, and fostering open communication. These approaches create a supportive environment in which individuals, especially children, can address their addiction and regain control over their technology usage. By combining these strategies with professional help when necessary, parents can guide their children toward a healthier and more balanced relationship with social media and technology.

6

THE 7-DAY ACTION PLAN

In the fast-paced and digitally driven world we live in, maintaining healthy family dynamics and ensuring responsible social media use among children can be a challenging task. The sixth chapter of our guide, titled "The 7-Day Action Plan," serves as a roadmap for parents to navigate this complex landscape. This chapter aims to provide parents with a practical, step-by-step plan for implementing social media boundaries and fostering healthier family dynamics. In this overview, we will discuss the purpose of the chapter and the significance of adopting a structured approach in today's digital age.

DAY 1: ASSESSING CURRENT SOCIAL MEDIA USAGE

Importance of Evaluation

The first step in our 7-Day Action Plan focuses on assessing the current state of social media usage within the family. This step is crucial for several reasons, emphasizing the importance of evaluation and its impact on relationships and family dynamics.

Awareness of Habits

Evaluating current social media usage brings awareness to family members about their digital habits. It allows parents and children to recognize how much time they spend on social media and whether it aligns with their goals and priorities.

Understanding the Impact

Assessment enables family members to understand the impact of excessive social media use on their lives. It sheds light on how it affects relationships, communication, and overall family dynamics.

Setting a Baseline

Assessment establishes a baseline for measuring progress. It helps identify areas that need improvement and provides a starting point for implementing changes.

Open Communication

Evaluating social media usage encourages open communication within the family. It promotes discussions about the role of technology, individual concerns, and collective goals related to digital device usage.

Informed Decision-Making

By evaluating their current habits, parents and children can make informed decisions about the changes they want to implement. It helps clarify what is and isn't working, guiding future strategies.

Strategies for Tracking and Monitoring

To assess current social media usage effectively, parents can employ practical strategies for tracking and monitoring.

Here are some strategies for parents to consider:

Use Screen Time Tracking Apps

Screen time tracking apps are valuable tools for monitoring social media usage. These apps provide detailed reports on the amount of time spent on various apps and websites. Parents can install such apps on their children's devices and set limits based on their findings.

Create Usage Logs

Encourage family members to create usage logs, documenting their daily social media activities. This includes noting the platforms they use, the time spent, and the purpose (e.g., communication, entertainment, information). Logs can be maintained for a week to capture typical patterns.

Conduct Family Meetings

Hold family meetings to discuss social media usage openly. Create a safe and non-judgmental space for everyone to share their experiences and concerns. Use these discussions to gather insights into each family member's perspective.

Surveys and Questionnaires

Design surveys or questionnaires that family members can fill out anonymously. These can include questions about the perceived impact of social media on their lives, feelings of addiction, and personal goals regarding screen time.

Collaborative Tracking

Consider collaborative tracking, where family members collectively monitor each other's screen time. This approach promotes accountability and encourages mutual support in reducing excessive usage.

Set Clear Objectives

Before beginning the assessment, set clear objectives for what you want to achieve through the evaluation process. Define specific questions you aim to answer, such as "How much time is spent on social media daily?" or "In what ways has social media affected family interactions?"

Reflect on Impact

Encourage family members to reflect on the observed impact of excessive social media use. This reflection can encompass emotional, psychological, and relational aspects. Ask questions like "How does excessive social media use make you feel?" or "Have you noticed any changes in our family dynamics?"

Keep a Journal

Invite family members to keep journals where they record their thoughts and emotions related to social media usage. Journals can serve as personal records of their experiences and contribute to a deeper understanding of the effects of technology on their lives.

Seek External Input

Consider seeking input from external sources, such as therapists or counselors specializing in digital addiction. Their assessments and recommendations can provide valuable insights into the family's situation.

Set Time Frames

Establish time frames for tracking and monitoring. Decide how long the assessment period will last (e.g., one week) and when you will reconvene to discuss the findings.

Maintain Privacy and Trust

Ensure that monitoring efforts respect individual privacy and build trust within the family. Emphasize that the purpose of evaluation is to improve family dynamics, not to invade personal space.

Compare Expectations with Reality

Encourage family members to compare their expectations regarding social media usage with the reality they observe during the assessment. This can highlight discrepancies and motivate them to make changes.

Use Data Visualization

Visualize the data collected during the assessment period. Create charts or graphs that illustrate screen time patterns and their impact on daily life. Visual representations can make the information more accessible and actionable.

Day 1 of the 7-Day Action Plan focuses on assessing current social media usage within the family. Evaluation is essential for raising awareness, understanding the impact of digital habits, and setting the stage for meaningful change. Practical strategies, such as using screen time tracking apps, creating usage logs, and maintaining open communication, empower parents and children to gather valuable insights into their digital behavior. This step serves as a foundation for the subsequent days of the action plan, where specific actions will be taken to improve family dynamics and promote responsible social media use.

DAY 2: ESTABLISHING HOUSE RULES AND CONSEQUENCES

Day 2 of our 7-Day Action Plan marks a critical juncture in our journey toward responsible social media usage within the family. This day is dedicated to the process of setting clear house rules regarding social media usage and establishing consequences for any rule violations. We will explore the significance of this process, provide guidance on determining age-appropriate screen time limits, and discuss strategies for enforcing rules consistently and fairly.

Process of Setting Clear Rules

Importance of the Rule-Setting Process

The process of setting clear and effective house rules regarding social media usage is a vital aspect of responsible digital parenting. It serves as the foundation for fostering a healthy relationship with technology within the family. Let's delve into the importance of this process and how it can be approached:

Promoting Responsibility and Accountability

The rule-setting process encourages responsibility and accountability among family members, especially children and adolescents. It involves them in decisions related to their digital habits, helping them understand the importance of responsible technology use.

Aligning with Family Values

This process allows families to align their rules with their core values. It prompts discussions about what the family values most and how technology can be integrated into those values.

Fostering Communication

Engaging in the rule-setting process fosters open communication within the family. It provides a platform for family members to express their thoughts, concerns, and expectations regarding social media usage.

Tailoring Rules to Individual Needs

Each family member may have unique needs and preferences when it comes to technology use. The rule-setting process enables customization of rules to meet individual requirements while maintaining a collective framework.

Avoiding Ambiguity

By involving all family members in rule setting, ambiguity and misunderstandings are minimized. Everyone is clear about what is expected, reducing the chances of conflicts arising from unclear guidelines.

Age-Appropriate Screen Time Limits

When setting rules, consider age-appropriate screen time limits. Guidelines provided by reputable sources, such as the American Academy of Pediatrics, can serve as a helpful reference. These limits are generally based on age groups:

Children under 2 years

No screen time (except video chatting).

Children aged 2 to 5 years

Limit screen time to one hour per day of high-quality programming, preferably with co-viewing.

Children aged 6 years and older

Establish consistent limits on screen time while ensuring that it does not interfere with adequate sleep, physical activity, and other healthy behaviors.

Involving Children in the Rule-Making Process

Involving children in the rule-making process is essential to ensure their active participation and understanding. Here are strategies for parents to engage their children in this crucial process:

Age-Appropriate Discussions

Tailor discussions to be age-appropriate. Younger children may require simpler explanations and rules, while adolescents can engage in more complex conversations about digital responsibility.

Collaborative Decision-Making

Encourage collaboration by allowing children to have a say in establishing rules. Ask for their input and consider their suggestions when crafting guidelines.

Set Expectations Clearly

Communicate expectations clearly to children. Use straightforward language and examples that they can relate to their own experiences.

Explain the 'Why'

Explain the reasons behind the rules. Help children understand the potential consequences of excessive screen time, the importance of balance, and the impact on their well-being.

Negotiate within Boundaries

While involving children, establish non-negotiable boundaries. Certain rules, particularly those related to safety, may not be open for negotiation.

Create a Family Technology Contract

Consider creating a family technology contract. This document outlines the agreed-upon rules, consequences for rule violations, and responsibilities for both parents and children.

Regularly Review and Revise

The rule-setting process is not static. Periodically review and revise rules as children grow and family dynamics change.

Ensure that the rules remain relevant and effective.

Establishing Consequences

Importance of Establishing Consequences

Establishing consequences for violating social media rules is a critical aspect of responsible digital parenting. Consequences serve several important purposes within the family:

Accountability

Consequences hold family members accountable for their actions. They reinforce the idea that rules are not arbitrary but have real-world implications.

Learning Opportunity

Consequences provide valuable learning opportunities. They allow individuals to understand the direct relationship between their actions and the resulting outcomes.

Consistency

Consistently enforcing consequences demonstrates that rules are applied fairly and without bias. It reinforces the idea that everyone is subject to the same rules.

Encouraging Responsibility

Consequences encourage responsibility by teaching that responsible behavior leads to positive outcomes, while irresponsible behavior results in negative consequences.

Promoting Communication

Consequences often spark important conversations within the family. When applied, they provide opportunities to discuss the reasons behind the rules and the importance of adhering to them.

Strategies for Enforcing Rules Consistently and Fairly

To ensure that rules are enforced consistently and fairly, parents can employ various strategies:

Clearly Define Consequences

Clearly define the consequences for rule violations. Ensure that family members are aware of what to expect when rules are not followed.

Link Consequences to Violations

Establish a direct link between consequences and specific rule violations. Make it clear which rule was broken and why the consequence is being applied.

Be Consistent

Consistency is crucial in rule enforcement. Ensure that consequences are applied consistently to all family members. Avoid making exceptions.

Maintain a Calm and Neutral Tone

When addressing rule violations, maintain a calm and neutral tone. Avoid escalating conflicts by yelling or becoming overly emotional.

Use Progressive Discipline

Consider using progressive discipline. Start with mild consequences for minor violations and escalate to more significant consequences for repeated or severe infractions.

Encourage Self-Reflection

Encourage family members to reflect on their actions and consequences. This promotes personal responsibility and understanding of the connection between behavior and outcomes.

Allow for Discussion

While consequences should be applied, allow for discussions afterward. Use these opportunities to explain the reasons behind the rules and consequences and listen to family members' perspectives.

Reiterate the Importance of Rules

Periodically remind family members of the importance of rules and consequences. Reinforce that these guidelines exist to create a safe and balanced digital environment.

Model Responsible Behavior

Parents should model responsible behavior by adhering to the rules themselves. This sets a positive example for children to follow.

Encourage Accountability

Encourage family members to take accountability for their actions and consequences. This helps foster a sense of responsibility and ownership.

Review and Adjust Consequences

Just as with rules, consequences may need periodic review and adjustment. Ensure that they remain effective and aligned with the family's goals.

Day 2 of our 7-Day Action Plan focuses on the crucial processes of setting clear rules and consequences regarding social media usage within the family. By involving all family members, defining expectations, and aligning rules with family values, parents create a structured framework that promotes responsible technology use. Establishing consequences reinforces accountability, encourages responsibility, and ensures that rules are enforced consistently and fairly. This step sets the stage for the subsequent days of the action plan, where further strategies will be implemented to achieve a balanced and harmonious relationship with technology within the family.

DAY 3: COMMUNICATING THE NEW BOUNDARIES TO CHILDREN

On the third day of our 7-Day Action Plan, we delve into the crucial process of communicating the new social media boundaries to children. This step is essential for creating a shared understanding of the rules, fostering cooperation, and addressing potential resistance. In this comprehensive guide, we will explore the importance of open communication, provide practical techniques for explaining the rules, and discuss strategies for navigating potential resistance or pushback from children.

Importance of Open Communication

Significance of Open and Honest Communication

Open and honest communication with children about the new social media boundaries is paramount for several reasons. It plays a central role in ensuring that the rules are understood and embraced within the family dynamic:

Fostering Understanding

Open communication allows parents to explain the reasons behind the rules clearly. When children understand the purpose and necessity of the boundaries, they are more likely to comply willingly.

Building Trust

Transparent communication builds trust between parents and children. When children feel that their voices are heard and their opinions are considered, they are more likely to trust their parents' judgment.

Promoting Cooperation

Effective communication fosters a sense of cooperation. When children understand that the rules are in place to benefit them and the family, they are more likely to adhere to them willingly.

Encouraging Responsibility

Open discussions about rules encourage children to take responsibility for their actions. They learn that their behavior has consequences and that they have a role in adhering to the established boundaries.

Addressing Concerns

Communication provides a platform for children to express their concerns and ask questions. It allows parents to address any misunderstandings or fears and to provide reassurance.

Techniques for Explaining the Rules

Practical Techniques for Parents

Explaining the new social media rules to children requires parents to employ practical techniques that facilitate understanding and cooperation. Here are some techniques that can be effective:

Age-Appropriate Discussions

Tailor discussions to be age-appropriate. Younger children may require simpler explanations, while older adolescents can engage in more complex conversations about digital responsibility.

Use Real-Life Examples

Illustrate the reasons behind the rules with real-life examples. Share stories or anecdotes that highlight the potential consequences of irresponsible social media usage.

Relate to Their Interests

Connect the rules to your children's interests and concerns. Show them how responsible technology use aligns with their hobbies, friendships, and overall well-being.

Encourage Questions

Create an environment where children feel comfortable asking questions. Encourage them to seek clarification on any aspects of the rules they do not understand.

Empathize with Their Feelings

Acknowledge and empathize with your children's feelings. Recognize that they may have mixed emotions about the rules, and validate their concerns.

Be Patient and Calm

Maintain patience and a calm demeanor during discussions. Avoid becoming defensive or confrontational if your children express reservations or disagree with certain rules. *Collaborative Decision-Making*

Involve children in decision-making when appropriate. Seek their input on rules that directly affect them, such as screen time limits or tech-free zones.

Use Visual Aids

Visual aids, such as charts or diagrams, can help simplify complex concepts. Create visuals that illustrate the rules and their benefits.

Highlight the Positive

Emphasize the positive aspects of the rules. Discuss how responsible technology use can lead to better concentration, more meaningful interactions, and a healthier balance between online and offline life.

Be Consistent in Messaging

Ensure that both parents present a united front when explaining the rules. Consistency in messaging helps avoid confusion and mixed signals.

Navigating Potential Resistance

Strategies for Addressing Resistance

It is common for children to exhibit resistance or pushback when confronted with new social media boundaries. Parents can employ strategies to navigate this resistance and ensure a collaborative implementation of the rules:

Listen Actively

Listen actively to your children's concerns and objections. Give them an opportunity to express their thoughts and feelings without interruption.

Validate Their Feelings

Validate your children's feelings by acknowledging their emotions and perspectives. Let them know that their feelings are valid even if you do not agree with their objections.

Explain the 'Why'

Reiterate the reasons behind the rules. Explain the potential bene-fits and how the rules contribute to their wellbeing and family harmony.

Offer Choices within Boundaries

Provide children with choices within the established boundaries. This empowers them to make decisions while still adhering to the rules.

Negotiate When Appropriate

Be open to negotiation when it is reasonable. Some rules may be open for discussion and adaptation based on your children's feedback and maturity level.

Set Expectations

Clearly communicate your expectations regarding rule compliance. Let your children know what consequences may follow if rules are consistently violated.

Be Patient and Consistent

Maintain patience and consistency in enforcing the rules. Children may need time to adjust to the new boundaries, and consistent enforcement reinforces their importance.

Offer Support

Offer your support and guidance in adhering to the rules. Show that you are willing to help them navigate challenges and find alternatives to excessive screen time.

Lead by Example

Model responsible technology use by adhering to the rules yourself. Children are more likely to follow rules when they see their parents doing the same.

Monitor Progress

Regularly monitor progress and assess whether the rules are achieving their intended outcomes. Be open to adjusting rules as needed based on the family's experiences.

Day 3 of our 7-Day Action Plan focuses on communicating the new social media boundaries to children, a critical step in fostering responsible technology use within the family. Open and honest communication is essential for building understanding, cooperation, and trust. By employing practical techniques for explaining the rules, parents can ensure that children grasp the reasons behind the boundaries. Additionally, strategies for navigating potential resistance help parents address objections and foster a collaborative approach to rule implementation. This step paves the way for the subsequent days of the action plan, where further strategies will be implemented to achieve a balanced and harmonious relationship with technology within the family.

DAY 4: IMPLEMENTING TECH-FREE ZONES AND QUALITY BONDING TIME

Day 4 of our 7-Day Action Plan is dedicated to implementing tech-free zones and carving out quality bonding time within the family. In today's digital age, it is crucial to establish spaces and moments where technology takes a back seat, fostering face-to-face interaction and strengthening familial connections. This day's guide will provide strategies for identifying tech-free zones, creating opportunities for quality bonding time, and emphasizing the importance of parental leadership in this endeavor.

Identifying Tech-Free Zones

Strategies for Designating Tech-Free Zones

Designating specific areas or times in the home as techfree zones is a deliberate step toward reducing screen time and promoting genuine human interaction. Here are strategies to identify and implement these zones effectively:

Define the Purpose

Start by defining the purpose of tech-free zones. Consider what you want to achieve by designating certain spaces or times as device-free. Common goals include improving communication, fostering connection, and reducing distractions. *Involve the Family*

Involve all family members in the discussion and decision-making process. Seek their input on where and when tech-free zones should be established. Encourage them to share their thoughts on the benefits of such zones.

Designate Specific Areas

Identify specific areas in the home where technology use is not permitted. Common tech-free zones include:

Dining Area

Make meal times device-free to encourage family members to connect over shared meals.

Bedrooms

Create a rule that bedrooms are tech-free zones, promoting better sleep and personal space.

Living Room

Designate the living room as a space for face-to-face interaction, reading, or relaxation without screens.

Set Tech-Free Times

Establish specific times during the day or week when technology is put aside in favor of other activities. For example, designate certain hours in the evening as tech-free family time.

Create Visual Reminders

Use visual cues to reinforce tech-free zones. Post signs or stickers in designated areas to remind family members of the rule. Visual reminders are especially helpful for younger children.

Lead by Example

Parents should lead by example in adhering to tech-free zone rules. When children see their parents prioritizing face-toface interaction over screens, they are more likely to do the same.

Explain the Benefits

Communicate the benefits of tech-free zones to your family. Discuss how these zones enhance communication, reduce distractions, and create opportunities for meaningful interactions.

Gradual Implementation

If tech-free zones are new to your family, consider a gradual implementation. Start with a few specific areas or times and gradually expand as everyone becomes accustomed to the concept.

Regular Check-Ins

Hold regular family meetings to check in on how techfree zones are working. Encourage family members to share their experiences and suggest improvements or adjustments.

Flexibility when Needed

While it is important to have tech-free zones, there may be exceptions when technology use is necessary, such as for work or school. Be flexible and make exceptions when needed while maintaining the overall rule.

Strategies for Quality Bonding Time

Suggestions for Creating Quality Bonding Time

In addition to tech-free zones, creating opportunities for quality bonding time is essential for strengthening family relationships.

Here are suggestions for fostering such moments within the family:

Family Dinners

Regular family dinners provide an excellent opportunity for bonding. Set a rule that meals are enjoyed together without screens. Use this time for conversation, sharing stories, and connecting.

Game Nights

Designate a specific evening each week as game night. Play board games, card games, or engage in video game-free gaming experiences that encourage interaction and friendly competition.

Outdoor Activities

Plan outdoor activities that the family can enjoy together. These might include hiking, biking, picnics, or simply going for a walk in the neighborhood. Outdoor experiences provide a break from screens and encourage physical activity.

Movie or TV Nights

While screen time should be limited, occasional movie or TV nights can be a fun family activity. Choose a film or show that everyone can enjoy and watch together, complete with popcorn and snacks.

Arts and Crafts

Engage in creative activities like arts and crafts. Set aside time for family art projects, painting, or crafting. Encourage children to express themselves through art.

Cooking Together

Involve family members in meal preparation. Cooking together fosters collaboration and allows everyone to contribute to the meal. It's also an opportunity to share culinary traditions and favorite recipes.

Volunteer as a Family

Participating in volunteer activities as a family is a meaningful way to bond while making a positive impact on the community. Choose volunteer opportunities that align with your family's interests and values.

Storytelling Time

Allocate time for storytelling. Encourage family members to share stories from their lives, childhood memories, or imaginative tales. Storytelling promotes communication and creativity.

Tech-Free Weekends

Consider implementing tech-free weekends periodically. During these weekends, digital devices are put aside in favor of engaging in face-to-face activities and quality time together.

Plan Family Outings

Organize outings to places of interest, such as museums, parks, zoos, or historical sites. Exploring new places together can be an enriching experience that creates lasting memories.

Celebrate Achievements

Celebrate each other's achievements and milestones as a family. Acknowledge academic accomplishments, personal goals, or special occasions together.

Share Family Traditions

Share and uphold family traditions, whether they involve holidays, cultural celebrations, or unique customs. These traditions create a sense of belonging and continuity.

Emphasizing Parental Leadership

One of the key elements in successfully implementing tech-free zones and quality bonding time is parental leadership.

Parents must lead by example in prioritizing device-free time and actively participating in family activities. Here's why parental leadership is crucial:

Role Modeling

Parents serve as role models for their children. When parents demonstrate their commitment to tech-free zones and quality bonding time, children are more likely to follow suit.

Influence and Guidance

Parents have a significant influence on their children's behaviors and habits. By actively participating in family activities, parents provide guidance and structure.

Strengthening Connection

Parental involvement in family activities strengthens the parent-child connection. It fosters trust, communication, and a sense of togetherness.

Consistency

Parental consistency in adhering to rules and participating in tech-free zones and quality bonding time reinforces the importance of these activities.

Creating Positive Memories

Quality time spent with parents creates positive memories that children carry into adulthood. These memories shape their understanding of family and relationships.

Teaching Prioritization

Parental leadership teaches children the importance of prioritizing family and human interaction over digital distractions.

Day 4 of our 7-Day Action Plan focuses on the implementation of tech-free zones and quality bonding time within the family. By designating specific areas or times as techfree zones and creating opportunities for meaningful bonding experiences, parents can foster stronger connections and reduce screen time. Emphasizing parental leadership in adhering to these rules and actively participating in family activities sets a positive example for children to follow. This step lays the foundation for the subsequent days of the action plan, where further strategies will be implemented to achieve a balanced and harmonious relationship with technology within the family.

DAY 5: PRACTICING ACTIVE LISTENING AND OPEN COMMUNICATION

Day 5 of our 7-Day Action Plan is dedicated to the essential practices of active listening and open communication within the family. These fundamental skills are instrumental in building strong connections with children, fostering understanding, and nurturing healthy parent-child relationships. In this guide, we will explore the significance of active listening, provide practical techniques for enhancing active listening skills, discuss the creation of a safe and non-judgmental environment, and offer strategies for fostering open communication within the family.

Significance of Active Listening

Exploration of the Importance of Active Listening

Active listening is a cornerstone of effective communication and plays a central role in building strong connections with children. It involves giving full attention to the speaker, understanding their perspective, and responding thoughtfully. The significance of active listening in parent-child relationships cannot be overstated:

Fostering Understanding

Active listening promotes a deep understanding of a child's thoughts, feelings, and concerns. It allows parents to grasp the underlying emotions and motivations behind what their child is saying.

Strengthening Trust

When children feel heard and understood, they are more likely to trust their parents. Trust is a foundational element of any strong parent-child relationship.

Validation of Feelings

Active listening validates a child's feelings and experiences. It acknowledges that their emotions are real and important, even if they differ from the parent's perspective.

Building Empathy

By actively listening, parents develop empathy for their children's experiences. They gain insight into the challenges and joys their children face, strengthening their ability to relate to them.

Encouraging Openness

Active listening creates an environment where children feel safe to express themselves openly. They are more likely to share their thoughts and concerns when they believe their words are valued.

Conflict Resolution

Active listening is a crucial skill in resolving conflicts within the family. It allows parents to understand the root causes of disagreements and work toward mutually agreeable solutions.

Practical Techniques for Enhancing Active Listening Skills

Enhancing active listening skills is a continuous process that involves honing certain techniques and approaches. Here are practical techniques for parents to become better active listeners:

Give Your Full Attention

When your child is speaking, give them your undivided attention. Put away distractions such as phones, tablets, or other devices, and make eye contact to convey your focus.

Show Empathy

Try to see the situation from your child's perspective. Show empathy by acknowledging their feelings and demonstrating that you care about how they are experiencing a situation.

Avoid Interrupting

Resist the urge to interrupt or offer immediate solutions when your child is speaking. Allow them to express themselves fully before responding.

Use Non-Verbal Cues

Use non-verbal cues such as nodding, smiling, and mirroring their emotions to signal that you are engaged in the conversation.

Reflect and Paraphrase

Reflect back what your child has said in your own words. This not only shows that you are actively listening but also helps clarify any misunderstandings.

Ask Open-Ended Questions

Encourage further discussion by asking open-ended questions that require more than a simple "yes" or "no" response. These questions invite your child to share more details and thoughts.

Validate Feelings

Validate your child's feelings by acknowledging them. Say things like, "I understand that you're feeling frustrated" or "It sounds like you had a great time today."

Avoid Judgment

Reserve judgment and criticism during the conversation. Create a safe space for your child to express themselves without fear of negative reactions.

Be Patient

Some children may take time to express themselves fully or may struggle to find the right words. Be patient and give them the space they need to communicate.

Encourage Expression

Encourage your child to express their thoughts and feelings. Let them know that you are there to listen and support them, no matter what they have to say.

Creating a Safe Environment

Discussion on Creating a Safe and Non-Judgmental Environment

Creating a safe and non-judgmental environment is essential for children to feel comfortable expressing their thoughts and feelings openly. Here's why this environment is crucial:

Emotional Safety

Children need to feel emotionally safe within their family. They should know that they can share their concerns, even if they are uncertain or anxious about how they will be received.

Trust Building

An environment of trust is built on mutual respect and acceptance. When children feel safe, they are more likely to trust their parents and share their experiences.

Healthy Communication

A safe environment fosters healthy communication patterns. It encourages open dialogue and minimizes the fear of criticism or judgment.

Emotional Growth

Children's emotional growth is nurtured in a safe and non-judgmental space. They can explore their emotions, learn to express themselves, and develop coping strategies.

Techniques for Fostering Open Communication

Fostering open communication within the family requires deliberate effort and specific techniques. Here are strategies for creating a safe and non-judgmental environment and encouraging open communication:

Listen Without Judgment

Avoid passing judgment or criticism when your child shares their thoughts or feelings. Create a space where they can express themselves freely.

Be Approachable

Make an effort to be approachable and available when your child wants to talk. Let them know that you are there to listen and support them, no matter the topic.

Respect Privacy

Respect your child's privacy, especially as they grow older. Allow them to share information at their own pace and avoid invading their personal space.

Use Encouraging Language

Use encouraging language that promotes open communication. Phrases like "I'm here for you" or "Tell me more" can invite further discussion.

Avoid Overreacting

Try to remain calm and composed, even if your child shares something unexpected or challenging. Overreacting can discourage future communication.

Set Aside Quality Time

Allocate quality one-on-one time with each child to foster individual communication. This creates opportunities for deeper conversations and bonding.

Encourage Journaling

Suggest journaling as a way for children to express their thoughts and feelings, especially if they find it challenging to verbalize them.

Create a Family Ritual

Establish a family ritual, such as a weekly family meeting, where everyone can openly discuss concerns, achievements, and plans.

Validate Their Perspectives

Even if you don't agree with your child's perspective, validate their right to have their own opinions and feelings. This fosters respect for differences.

Provide Support

Let your child know that you are there to support them, whether they are sharing joyful moments or facing challenges. Offer guidance and reassurance.

Day 5 of our 7-Day Action Plan underscores the importance of active listening and open communication in building strong connections with children. Active listening fosters understanding, trust, and empathy, while open communication creates a safe and non-judgmental environment for children to express themselves. By practicing these essential skills and employing the suggested techniques, parents can nurture healthy parent-child relationships and encourage their children to communicate openly. This step sets the stage for the remaining days of the action plan, where further strategies will be implemented to achieve a balanced and harmonious relationship with technology within the family.

DAY 6: ENGAGING IN SHARED ACTIVITIES AND HOBBIES

Benefits of Shared Activities

Engaging in shared activities and hobbies as a family is a powerful way to strengthen relationships and create lasting bonds. These shared experiences offer numerous benefits for family members of all ages. Here, we highlight the advantages of participating in shared activities and explore different types of activities that families can enjoy together.

Quality Bonding

Shared activities provide dedicated time for family members to connect and bond in a relaxed and enjoyable setting. They create opportunities for meaningful interactions and conversations.

Strengthening Relationships

Engaging in activities together fosters a sense of togetherness and unity within the family. It reinforces the idea that the family is a team that supports and enjoys one another's company.

Creating Lasting Memories

Shared activities often result in cherished memories that family members can look back on with fondness. These experiences become part of the family's history and narrative.

Enhancing Communication

During shared activities, family members communicate, collaborate, and solve problems together. This enhances communication skills and the ability to work as a team.

Reducing Screen Time

Many shared activities involve minimal or no screen time, providing a break from digital devices and encouraging face-to-face interactions.

Building Tradition

Engaging in specific activities as a family can become a cherished tradition. These traditions contribute to a sense of continuity and belonging within the family.

Exploring Interests

Shared activities allow family members to explore new interests and passions together. This can lead to the discovery of hidden talents and shared hobbies.

Stress Reduction

Participating in enjoyable activities can serve as a stress reliever for both children and parents. It offers an opportunity to unwind and have fun together.

Types of Activities

Outdoor Adventures

Outdoor activities such as hiking, biking, camping, or nature walks are great for connecting with nature and each other.

Arts and Crafts

Engage in creative endeavors like painting, drawing, crafting, or DIY projects. These activities encourage selfexpression and creativity.

Cooking and Baking

Cooking meals or baking treats together can be a fun and delicious way to bond as a family. Everyone can take on different roles in the kitchen.

Board Games and Puzzles

Board games, card games, and puzzles offer opportunities for friendly competition, strategic thinking, and laughter.

Sports and Physical Activities

Play sports like soccer, basketball, or frisbee in the backyard or at a nearby park. Physical activities promote fitness and teamwork.

Gardening

Cultivating a garden together allows family members to nurture plants, learn about nature, and enjoy the outdoors.

Music and Dance

Explore music through singing, dancing, or learning to play musical instruments together. Music fosters creativity and self-expression.

Reading

Choose a book to read as a family and have regular reading sessions where everyone can discuss the story's progress.

Volunteer Work

Participate in volunteer activities or community service as a family. This instills a sense of social responsibility and empathy in children.

Identifying Children's Interests

Identifying and nurturing children's interests is essential when it comes to selecting shared activities and hobbies. Understanding their passions and preferences can help parents find common ground for enjoyable family experiences. Here are practical suggestions on how parents can identify their children's interests and create meaningful shared activities:

Observe and Listen

Pay attention to what your children naturally gravitate toward. Observe their playtime activities, hobbies, and the topics they like to discuss. Listen to their conversations and questions.

Encourage Exploration

Provide opportunities for your children to explore various activities and interests. Take them to museums, art galleries, parks, or sports events to expose them to different experiences.

Ask Open-Ended Questions

Engage your children in conversations about their interests by asking open-ended questions. For example, "What do you enjoy doing in your free time?" or "What kinds of activities make you the happiest?"

Be Supportive

When your children express an interest in something, be supportive and encouraging. Show genuine enthusiasm for their pursuits, even if it's something you're not familiar with.

Try New Things Together

Explore new activities together as a family. This can include signing up for a class or workshop related to a particular interest your child has shown.

Adapt and Evolve

Children's interests can change over time. Stay open to their evolving passions and be willing to adapt shared activities accordingly.

Create a Hobby Space

Designate a space in your home where children can pursue their interests. This could be an art corner, a music nook, or a mini sports area.

Encourage Peer Interaction

Encourage your children to interact with peers who share similar interests. Playdates or group activities can further nurture their hobbies.

Celebrate Achievements

Celebrate your children's achievements and milestones related to their interests. Acknowledge their efforts and successes.

Set Realistic Expectations

While it's important to support your children's interests, also set realistic expectations. Not every interest will become a lifelong passion, and that's okay.

Versatility of Shared Activities

One of the remarkable aspects of shared activities is their versatility. They can adapt to the interests and ages of family members, making them accessible and enjoyable for everyone. Whether it's exploring nature, engaging in creative pursuits, or participating in physical activities, shared activities provide a common ground for connection and enjoyment. The key is to remain open to trying new things and to prioritize the quality of time spent together as a family.

Day 6 of our 7-Day Action Plan highlights the importance of engaging in shared activities and hobbies as a means of strengthening family relationships. These activities offer numerous benefits, from quality bonding and communication to reducing screen time and building traditions. By identifying and nurturing children's interests, parents can tailor shared activities to their unique passions and preferences.

The versatility of shared activities ensures that families can find enjoyable experiences that cater to the interests and ages of all family members. This step sets the stage for the final day of the action plan, where we will implement strategies for establishing boundaries and balance in technology use within the family.

DAY 7: REFLECTION AND FOLLOW-UP STRATEGIES

Reflecting on the Process

As we reach the final day of our 7-Day Action Plan, it's time for parents to engage in reflection. Taking a moment to reflect on the progress made during this action plan is essential. This step encourages parents to recognize the positive changes observed in family dynamics and relationships as a result of implementing social media boundaries.

Encouragement for Parents to Reflect

Reflecting on the process allows parents to appreciate the journey they've undertaken to foster healthier relationships with technology in their family. Here are some key points to consider during this reflection:

Recognizing Achievements

Acknowledge the achievements and milestones reached during the 7-day action plan. Celebrate the positive changes and efforts made by both parents and children.

Assessing Challenges

Reflect on any challenges or difficulties faced along the way. Identify areas where further improvement or adjustments may be needed.

Observing Behavioral Changes

Pay attention to any notable behavioral changes in your children's screen time habits and overall well-being. Have there been improvements in their sleep, academic performance, or social interactions?

Family Bonding

Reflect on the quality of family bonding and communication that has occurred during shared activities and tech-free moments. Consider the impact of these interactions on family dynamics.

Personal Growth

Reflect on your own personal growth as a parent. Have you developed new skills or insights during this process? How has your relationship with your children evolved?

Discussion on the Positive Changes Observed

Encourage open discussions with your children about the positive changes observed during the 7-day action plan. Include them in the reflection process, as their input is valuable in understanding the impact of these changes on their lives. Here are some potential positive changes to discuss:

Improved Communication

Talk about how communication within the family has improved. Have there been more meaningful conversations or increased openness between family members?

Quality Time

Highlight the quality time spent together during shared activities and tech-free moments. Discuss the enjoyable experiences and memories created as a family.

Reduced Screen Time

Address the reduction in excessive screen time and the resulting benefits, such as improved sleep patterns, increased physical activity, and enhanced focus on academic tasks.

Behavioral Changes

Share any positive behavioral changes you've observed in your children, such as reduced social media preoccupation, increased engagement in other activities, or better time management.

Increased Awareness

Talk about the increased awareness of the impact of social media on well-being and relationships. Discuss how this awareness has influenced choices and habits.

Enhanced Family Bond

Emphasize the strengthened family bond and the importance of maintaining this connection. Share your appreciation for the effort put into creating a healthier digital balance.

Follow-Up Strategies

While the 7-Day Action Plan provides an excellent starting point for establishing social media boundaries and improving family dynamics, it's crucial to recognize that this is an ongoing process. To maintain the positive changes and continue fostering healthy relationships with technology, parents should implement follow-up strategies. These strategies involve ongoing communication and adaptation of rules based on family needs.

Introduction to Follow-Up Strategies

Follow-up strategies are designed to ensure that the progress made during the 7-day action plan is sustained in the long term. They help families maintain the established social media boundaries and adapt them as needed to accommodate changing circumstances. Here are key components of follow-up strategies:

Regular Family Check-Ins

Schedule regular family meetings or check-ins to discuss screen time habits, challenges, and successes. Encourage open dialogue and allow family members to voice their concerns or suggestions.

Monitor and Adjust

Continuously monitor screen time usage and its impact on family life. Be prepared to adjust rules and boundaries if necessary. Flexibility is essential as children grow and technology evolves.

Set Realistic Expectations

Establish realistic expectations for screen time limits and behavior. Ensure that rules are age-appropriate and align with the needs of each child.

Positive Reinforcement

Continue to provide positive reinforcement for adherence to social media boundaries. Reward children for responsible technology use and achieving personal goals.

Education and Awareness

Keep the family informed about the potential risks and benefits of social media and technology. Encourage responsible digital citizenship and critical thinking.

Role Modeling

Lead by example as parents by demonstrating responsible technology use and maintaining a healthy digital balance in your own lives.

Flexibility

Be flexible in your approach and willing to make adjustments based on individual circumstances. Each child may have unique needs and challenges.

Seek Professional Guidance

If necessary, seek professional guidance from therapists, counselors, or experts in technology addiction. They can provide valuable insights and support.

Maintain Shared Activities

Continue engaging in shared activities and hobbies as a family. These experiences strengthen bonds and provide alternatives to excessive screen time.

Stay Informed

Stay informed about the latest trends and issues related to technology and social media. Being aware of emerging challenges can help you address them proactively.

Ongoing Communication

Central to successful follow-up strategies is the importance of ongoing communication within the family. Maintain an environment where children feel comfortable discussing their experiences, challenges, and concerns related to technology. Encourage them to seek guidance and support from parents when needed.

Adaptation and Growth

Remember that family dynamics, technology, and children's needs will evolve over time. Adaptation is a natural part of the process. Be open to reassessing and modifying rules and boundaries to accommodate these changes while prioritizing the well-being of your children and the strength of your family connections.

As we conclude the 7-Day Action Plan, parents are encouraged to reflect on the progress achieved and the positive changes observed in family dynamics and relationships. This reflection sets the stage for implementing effective follow-up strategies that will help maintain the established social media boundaries and continue fostering healthy relationships with technology. The journey toward a balanced and harmonious digital life is ongoing, and with dedication and communication, families can thrive in the digital age while prioritizing their wellbeing and connection with one another.

7
ADDRESSING CHALLENGES AND RESISTANCE

Addressing Challenges in the Digital Age

Parenting in the digital age presents a unique set of challenges that previous generations did not have to navigate. The omnipresence of technology, the influence of social media, and the rapid evolution of digital devices have transformed the landscape of parenting. This chapter explores the multifaceted challenges parents encounter in the digital age, including resistance from children, managing peer pressure, and fostering healthy digital habits. By understanding and addressing these challenges, parents can navigate the complexities of raising digitally literate and responsible children.

The Digital Transformation

The digital transformation has revolutionized nearly every aspect of modern life, including how families communicate, learn, and entertain themselves. Children today grow up in a digital environment that offers unparalleled access to information, entertainment, and social connections. While this presents numerous opportunities, it also comes with challenges that parents must navigate.

Understanding the Challenges

To effectively address the challenges of parenting in a digital age, it is essential to understand the specific difficulties parents encounter:

Resistance and Pushback from Children

One of the most common challenges parents face is resistance and pushback from their children regarding screen time limits and digital boundaries. Children often see digital devices and social media as integral parts of their social lives and may resist efforts to reduce their screen time.

Managing Peer Pressure

Peer pressure has taken on a new dimension in the digital age. Children may feel pressured to conform to online trends, engage in risky behaviors, or spend excessive time on social media platforms due to the influence of their peers.

Fostering Healthy Digital Habits

Teaching children to develop healthy digital habits is essential for their well-being. This includes responsible screen time management, critical thinking about online content, and understanding the impact of their online actions.

Balancing Screen Time

Finding the right balance between screen time for educational purposes and recreational activities can be challenging. Parents must strike a balance that aligns with their family's values and goals.

Online Safety and Privacy

Ensuring online safety and privacy is a significant concern for parents. Children must be educated about the risks of sharing personal information online and the potential consequences of cyberbullying and online harassment.

Staying Informed

Keeping up with the latest digital trends and technologies can be overwhelming for parents. Staying informed is crucial to providing guidance and support to children in their digital journeys.

Addressing Resistance and Pushback

Understanding the Reasons

When children resist digital boundaries, it's essential to understand the underlying reasons for their resistance. They may perceive social media and screen time as a source of connection, entertainment, or identity development. Engage in open conversations to uncover their motivations.

Communication and Empathy

Effective communication is key to addressing resistance. Be empathetic and acknowledge your child's perspective. Show understanding and genuine interest in their online experiences. Avoid judgment and criticism, which can lead to further resistance.

Negotiation and Collaboration

Involve children in the decision-making process regarding digital boundaries. Negotiate and collaborate to find mutually acceptable solutions. By including them in the process, they may be more willing to adhere to the agreed-upon rules.

Setting Clear Expectations

Clearly articulate your expectations regarding screen time, online behavior, and digital boundaries. Make these expectations part of a family agreement or digital contract. Having concrete guidelines can reduce ambiguity and resistance.

Positive Reinforcement

Reinforce positive behaviors and responsible digital choices with praise and encouragement. Recognize and celebrate when your child follows the established rules. Positive reinforcement can motivate them to continue making responsible choices.

Modeling Behavior

Lead by example in demonstrating responsible digital behavior. Children are more likely to adopt healthy digital habits if they see their parents practicing them. Show that screen time is not just for children; adults also set limits and prioritize other activities.

Managing Peer Pressure

Open Discussions

Initiate open discussions about peer pressure and online trends. Encourage your child to share their experiences and concerns. Be a trusted source of guidance and support as they navigate peer influences in the digital world.

Critical Thinking Skills

Teach your child critical thinking skills to help them assess the legitimacy and safety of online content. Encourage them to question information, be discerning consumers of media, and recognize potential pitfalls.

Respectful Dissent

Empower your child to respectfully dissent from online pressures that go against their values or make them uncomfortable. Teach them that it is okay to say no to activities or trends that do not align with their beliefs.

Building Self-Esteem

Foster your child's self-esteem and self-confidence. Children with strong self-esteem are better equipped to resist negative peer pressure and make independent choices.

Monitoring and Guidance

Maintain an active role in monitoring your child's online interactions, especially in the early stages of their digital journey. Offer guidance on identifying and responding to peer pressure situations.

Fostering Healthy Digital Habits

Digital Literacy Education

Provide your child with digital literacy education that includes topics like online etiquette, privacy, and cyberbullying. Equip them with the knowledge and skills needed to navigate the digital world safely and responsibly.

Setting Screen Time Limits

Establish reasonable screen time limits that align with your family's values and priorities. Ensure that these limits allow for a balance between online and offline activities, including family time.

Encourage Offline Activities

Promote a variety of offline activities and interests to reduce reliance on screens. Encourage physical activity, hobbies, reading, and face-to-face interactions with friends and family.

Tech-Free Zones

Designate tech-free zones or times within your home to promote family interactions without digital distractions. Meals, family outings, and bedtime can be ideal times to disconnect from screens.

Open Communication

Maintain open lines of communication with your child about their online experiences. Encourage them to share any concerns, encounters with cyberbullying, or discomfort they may have online.

Consistent Enforcement

Consistency in enforcing digital rules and consequences is essential. Ensure that consequences for rule violations are fair, reasonable, and consistently applied.

Online Safety Measures

Implement online safety measures, such as privacy settings and content filters, to protect your child from harmful content and online threats. Regularly review and update these settings.

Collaboration with Schools

Collaborate with your child's school to promote responsible technology use. Stay informed about the school's policies on screen time and online safety.

Seeking Professional Guidance

If you encounter persistent challenges or concerns, do not hesitate to seek professional guidance from therapists, counselors, or experts specializing in child development and technology addiction.

Staying Informed

Continuous Learning

The digital landscape is ever-evolving, making continuous learning essential for parents. Stay informed about new technologies, social media platforms, and emerging digital trends.

Online Resources

Explore online resources, workshops, and courses that provide guidance on digital parenting. These resources can help you stay up-to-date and equipped to address digital challenges.

Parental Control Tools

Familiarize yourself with parental control tools and apps that can assist in monitoring and managing your child's online activities.

Support Networks

Join support networks or online communities of parents who face similar challenges. Sharing experiences and advice with other parents can be invaluable.

Parenting in the digital age is a journey filled with complexities and challenges. By understanding the reasons behind resistance, effectively communicating, and fostering healthy digital habits, parents can navigate these challenges with confidence. Additionally, addressing peer pressure, staying informed, and seeking professional guidance when needed are crucial components of successful digital parenting. Ultimately, the goal is to raise digitally responsible and resilient children who can thrive in the digital world while maintaining a healthy balance between online and offline life.

DEALING WITH PUSHBACK AND RESISTANCE FROM CHILDREN

Strategies for Handling Resistance

Dealing with pushback and resistance from children when implementing social media boundaries can be a challenging aspect of digital parenting. However, effective strategies can help parents address these issues in a constructive and supportive manner. In this section, we will discuss strategies for handling resistance and explore communication techniques to address concerns and objections.

Understanding the Reasons Behind Resistance

Before diving into specific strategies, it's crucial for parents to understand the reasons behind their child's resistance to social media boundaries. Common motivations for resistance include:

Desire for Independence

Adolescents, in particular, may resist rules as they seek independence and autonomy.

Peer Pressure

Children often want to fit in with their peers, and social media can be a significant platform for social interaction.

Fear of Missing Out (FOMO)

Children may worry about missing out on social events or trends if they are not actively engaged on social media.

Lack of Awareness

Some children may not fully grasp the potential risks associated with excessive screen time or inappropriate online behavior.

Open and Empathetic Communication

Effective communication is at the core of addressing resistance. Parents should create an environment where children feel comfortable expressing their concerns and opinions. Here are some communication techniques to consider:

Active Listening

Listen attentively to your child's perspective without interrupting or immediately offering solutions. Reflect back what they've said to show that you understand.

Empathy

Show empathy and understanding by acknowledging

your child's feelings and concerns. Empathy can help reduce defensiveness and open the door to more productive conversations.

Non-Judgmental Approach

Avoid criticizing or blaming your child for their resistance. Instead, focus on finding solutions together.

Ask Open-Ended Questions

Encourage your child to share their thoughts and feelings by asking open-ended questions. This promotes deeper conversations.

Validate Their Feelings

Let your child know that their feelings are valid, even if you don't necessarily agree with their perspective.

Collaborative Problem-Solving

Involving your child in the decision-making process regarding social media boundaries can foster a sense of ownership and cooperation. Here's how to approach collaborative problem-solving:

Family Meeting

Hold a family meeting to discuss digital rules and boundaries. Encourage everyone to contribute their ideas and concerns.

Establish Clear Expectations

Clearly articulate your expectations for social media use.

Share your concerns and explain the reasons behind the rules.

Negotiate and Compromise

Be willing to negotiate and find compromises that take into account both your child's desires and your concerns as a parent.

Create a Family Agreement

Consider creating a family agreement or digital contract that outlines the rules, consequences, and rewards. All family members can sign it to signify their commitment.

Flexibility

Be open to revisiting and adjusting rules as your child matures and circumstances change. Flexibility demonstrates that you are willing to adapt to their needs.

Role Modeling

Parents play a crucial role in shaping their children's attitudes and behaviors, including their approach to technology. To encourage responsible technology use, parents should lead by example:

Set Boundaries for Yourself

Show that screen time is not just a concern for children but for adults as well. Set your own boundaries and adhere to them.

Be Mindful of Screen Time

Demonstrate mindfulness in your screen time habits. Avoid constantly checking your phone or being glued to screens during family time.

Engage in Shared Activities

Prioritize shared family activities that do not involve screens. Show that you value face-to-face interactions.

Openly Discuss Your Challenges

Share your own struggles and challenges with technology. This can help your child understand that managing screen time is an ongoing effort for everyone.

Positive Reinforcement

Positive reinforcement is a powerful motivator for children. Acknowledge and reward responsible technology use and adherence to social media boundaries:

Praise and Encouragement

Offer praise and encouragement when your child follows the established rules. Recognize their efforts and successes.

Incentives

Consider offering incentives or rewards for responsible behavior, such as extra screen time on weekends or special privileges.

Natural Consequences

Allow natural consequences to unfold when rules are followed. For example, if your child manages their screen time well, they may have more free time for other activities they enjoy.

Seek Professional Guidance When Needed

If resistance persists and becomes a source of ongoing conflict, consider seeking professional guidance. Therapists, counselors, or experts in child development and technology addiction can provide valuable insights and strategies to address resistance effectively.

Encouraging Cooperation and Compromise

Encouraging cooperation and compromise between parents and children regarding social media rules is essential for creating a harmonious digital environment within the family. Practical examples and scenarios can help parents navigate challenging situations effectively.

Scenario: Negotiating Screen Time Limits

Challenge

Your child strongly opposes the screen time limits you've set, arguing that their friends get to use devices without restrictions.

Strategy

Hold a Discussion

Initiate a calm and respectful discussion with your child to understand their perspective. Ask open-ended questions like,

"Why do you think screen time limits are unfair?"

Listen Actively

Listen actively and empathetically to their concerns without interrupting. Acknowledge their desire for fairness and social interaction.

Explain the Reasons

Explain the reasons behind the screen time limits, such as the importance of balance, sleep quality, and maintaining offline relationships.

Negotiate

Offer to negotiate the limits together. Ask your child for their input on what they believe is a reasonable compromise.

Create a Screen Time Schedule

Collaboratively create a screen time schedule that takes into account both your concerns and your child's preferences.

Set Realistic Expectations

Ensure that the negotiated screen time limits are realistic and align with your family's values and goals.

Scenario: Resistance to Parental Monitoring

Challenge

Your teenager resists your efforts to monitor their online activities, viewing it as an invasion of privacy.

Strategy

Open Dialogue

Initiate an open dialogue about online safety and the importance of parental monitoring. Explain that monitoring is a way to ensure their safety.

Respect Privacy

Acknowledge their need for privacy and independence. Emphasize that monitoring is not about mistrust but about guidance and protection.

Transparency

Be transparent about the monitoring tools or apps you use and how they work. Encourage questions and discussion.

Set Boundaries

Establish clear boundaries regarding which aspects of their online life will be monitored and which will remain private. *Gradual Independence*

As your child demonstrates responsible online behavior and maturity, gradually reduce the level of monitoring, allowing them more independence.

Scenario: Peer Pressure to Share Inappropriate Content

Challenge

Your child's friends pressure them to share inappropriate content or engage in risky online behaviors.

Strategy

Educate About Consequences

Have an open and honest conversation about the potential consequences of sharing inappropriate content, including legal and reputational risks.

Discuss Peer Pressure

Teach your child to recognize and resist peer pressure, both online and offline. Share strategies for saying no assertively.

Digital Literacy

Provide guidance on digital literacy and responsible online behavior. Emphasize the importance of critical thinking and making informed choices.

Role-Play Scenarios

Practice role-playing scenarios with your child to help them build confidence in saying no to inappropriate requests from peers.

Encourage Reporting

Encourage your child to report any instances of peer pressure or bullying to a trusted adult, whether it occurs online or offline.

Scenario: Reluctance to Participate in Offline Activities

Challenge

Your child is resistant to participating in offline activities or spending quality time with the family because they prefer screen-based interactions.

Strategy

Explain the Benefits

Discuss the benefits of offline activities, such as physical health, creativity, and strengthened family bonds.

Offer Choices

Give your child choices for offline activities, allowing them to select activities that align with their interests.

Family Engagement

Engage the whole family in offline activities. Plan fun outings, game nights, or creative projects that everyone can enjoy together.

Gradual Transition

If your child is particularly attached to screens, implement a gradual transition by starting with short offline activities and gradually increasing their duration.

Lead by Example

Model offline engagement by participating enthusiastically in family activities. Your enthusiasm can be contagious.

Scenario: Addressing Sleep Disruption Due to LateNight Screen Use

Challenge

Your child resists turning off screens at bedtime, leading to sleep disruption and fatigue.

Strategy

Educate About Sleep

Explain the importance of quality sleep for physical and mental health, including academic performance and mood.

Set a Bedtime Routine

Establish a consistent bedtime routine that includes winding down without screens. Encourage relaxation activities like reading.

Device Charging

Implement a rule that devices must be charged outside the bedroom to prevent late-night screen use.

Collaborative Agreement

Involve your child in creating a bedtime agreement that outlines the steps to prepare for sleep, including when screens should be turned off.

Consequences

Clearly communicate consequences for not following the bedtime rules, such as reduced screen time the following day.

Dealing with pushback and resistance from children when implementing social media boundaries is a common challenge for parents in the digital age. However, by understanding the reasons behind resistance, practicing effective communication, encouraging cooperation and compromise, and addressing specific scenarios, parents can navigate these challenges successfully. The key is to create a supportive and open environment where children feel heard and understood while maintaining a balance between digital engagement and offline activities that promote overall well-being.

MANAGING PEER PRESSURE AND SOCIAL MEDIA INFLUENCE

Fostering Critical Thinking Skills

Fostering critical thinking skills in children is essential to help them navigate social pressures and online influences effectively. Critical thinking empowers children to evaluate information, make informed decisions, and resist negative online peer pressure. Here are tips for parents on fostering these skills:

Encourage Questioning

Parents can encourage their children to ask questions about what they encounter online. Encourage curiosity and the desire to seek more information.

Teach Media Literacy

Help children develop media literacy skills by teaching them to assess the credibility and reliability of online sources.

Discuss how to differentiate between fact and opinion, as well as the importance of verifying information before accepting it as truth.

Promote Skepticism

Teach children to be skeptical of sensationalist headlines, clickbait, and content that seems too good to be true.

Encourage them to fact-check information and seek multiple sources for confirmation.

Discuss Bias

Engage in conversations about bias in media and online content. Explain that different sources may have different perspectives and agendas.

Encourage children to critically analyze content that may be biased and consider alternative viewpoints.

Self-Esteem and Self-Worth

Fostering self-esteem and self-worth in children is crucial. Children with strong self-esteem are more likely to resist negative peer pressure, both online and offline.

Help your child build self-confidence by acknowledging their strengths, praising their efforts, and supporting their passions and interests.

Positive Online Identity

Encourage your child to develop a positive online identity based on their values and interests. Emphasize that they do not have to conform to negative online trends to gain acceptance.

Educating About Risks and Consequences

Educating children about the potential risks and consequences of excessive social media use is essential for their safety and well-being. Parents can employ various strategies to impart this knowledge effectively:

Open Dialogue

Create an open and non-judgmental space for discussions about online risks and consequences. Encourage your child to share their experiences and concerns.

Age-Appropriate Conversations

Tailor conversations to your child's age and maturity level. Younger children may need simpler explanations, while older children can engage in more in-depth discussions.

Online Privacy

Teach your child about the importance of online privacy. Discuss the potential risks of sharing personal information and photos with strangers online.

Cyberbullying Awareness

Educate your child about cyberbullying, its forms, and its effects. Encourage them to report any instances of cyberbullying to a trusted adult.

Consequences of Oversharing

Discuss the consequences of oversharing on social media. Explain that once something is posted online, it can be challenging to control who sees it and how it may be used.

Digital Footprint

Help your child understand the concept of a digital footprint. Teach them that their online actions can have longterm consequences on their reputation and future opportunities.

Responsible Social Media Use

Emphasize responsible social media use, including respectful communication and refraining from sharing hurtful or inappropriate content.

Resisting Negative Online Peer Pressure

Teaching children how to resist negative online peer pressure is crucial for their well-being and safety. Parents can provide practical strategies and guidance to support their children in making independent and positive online choices:

Open Communication

Maintain open lines of communication with your child. Encourage them to share any instances of negative online peer pressure or uncomfortable situations.

Teach Assertiveness

Teach your child assertiveness skills to help them confidently say no to online pressures or requests that go against their values.

Role-play scenarios to practice assertive responses to peer pressure.

Discuss Boundaries

Help your child establish and communicate personal boundaries for online interactions. Explain that it is okay to set limits on what they are comfortable sharing or participating in.

Recognize Manipulation

Educate your child about manipulation tactics that may be used by peers online. Discuss the importance of recognizing when someone is trying to pressure or manipulate them.

Empower Independence

Encourage your child to trust their instincts and judgment. Remind them that it is acceptable to make independent decisions about online participation.

Supportive Friends

Encourage your child to surround themselves with friends who support and respect their boundaries. Discuss the importance of choosing friends who share similar values.

Reporting and Blocking

Teach your child how to report and block individuals

who engage in negative online behaviors. Ensure they understand that seeking help from a trusted adult is a responsible choice.

Self-Care

Emphasize the importance of self-care and mental wellbeing. Teach your child to recognize when online interactions become emotionally draining and when it's time to take a break.

Reinforce Online vs. Offline Values

Help your child understand that their values and principles should remain consistent both online and offline. Encourage them to stay true to themselves.

Managing peer pressure and social media influence is a critical aspect of parenting in the digital age. Fostering critical thinking skills, educating children about risks and consequences, and teaching them how to resist negative online peer pressure are vital components of helping children navigate the online world safely and responsibly. By providing guidance and maintaining open communication, parents can empower their children to make informed decisions and build a positive online presence while staying true to their values and principles.

SUPPORTING CHILDREN IN DEVELOPING HEALTHY DIGITAL HABITS

Setting Realistic and Achievable Goals

Setting realistic and achievable goals for screen time is a fundamental step in supporting children to develop healthy digital habits. It's essential for parents to understand the importance of balance and provide practical guidance on determining appropriate digital habits based on individual needs.

Understanding the Role of Goals

Parents should convey to their children that setting goals for screen time is not about restriction but about finding a healthy balance between online and offline activities.

Individualized Approach

Recognize that every child is different, and what constitutes a healthy digital habit may vary based on factors such as age, school requirements, and extracurricular activities.

Collaborative Goal-Setting

Involve your child in the goal-setting process. Ask them about their priorities and preferences when it comes to screen time.

Age-Appropriate Guidelines

Consider age-appropriate guidelines recommended by experts. For instance, the American Academy of Pediatrics provides screen time guidelines for different age groups.

Flexibility

Be flexible in adapting goals as your child's needs change. What works for a younger child may not be suitable for a teenager.

Monitor and Adjust

Continuously monitor your child's screen time and assess whether the goals set are realistic and achievable. Be willing to make adjustments as needed.

Rewards and Consequences

Implement a system of rewards and consequences to motivate your child to adhere to their screen time goals. Reward responsible use and enforce consequences for excessive use.

Encouraging Alternative Activities

Encouraging children to engage in alternative activities beyond screen time is vital for promoting a balanced and healthy lifestyle. Here are strategies for parents to consider:

Diverse Activities

Introduce your child to a variety of activities, both indoor and outdoor, that align with their interests. This may include sports, arts and crafts, cooking, reading, or exploring nature.

Family Involvement

Engage in activities as a family to make them more appealing. Family outings, game nights, or collaborative projects can be enjoyable and memorable experiences.

Screen-Free Zones

Designate specific areas or times in the home as screenfree zones or hours. For instance, the dining table can be a screen-free zone during meal times.

Hobbies and Passions

Encourage your child to discover and pursue their hobbies and passions. Whether it's playing a musical instrument, gardening, or coding, hobbies provide a sense of fulfillment.

Balancing Screen Time with Physical Activity

Emphasize the importance of physical activity.

Encourage your child to participate in sports or engage in regular physical exercise to maintain a healthy lifestyle.

Creative Outlets

Support your child's creativity by providing access to art supplies, musical instruments, or writing materials. Creative outlets can be a source of joy and self-expression.

Peer Interaction

Facilitate opportunities for your child to interact with peers in real-life settings. Playdates, group activities, and clubs can foster social connections outside of screens.

Importance of Parental Role Modeling

The role of parental role modeling in shaping children's digital habits cannot be overstated. Parents serve as powerful role models for their children's behavior, including their approach to technology and screens. Here are tips for parents on creating a supportive environment that fosters healthy digital habits:

Lead by Example

Demonstrate responsible and balanced screen time habits in your own life. Children are more likely to emulate behavior they observe in their parents.

Establish Family Rules

Create clear and consistent family rules regarding screen time. Enforce these rules for all family members, including adults.

Share Offline Interests

Share your offline interests and hobbies with your child.

Engage in activities that do not involve screens together.

Technology-Free Quality Time

Designate specific times for technology-free quality time as a family. This can include family dinners, board game nights, or outdoor adventures.

Open Communication

Maintain open communication with your child about digital habits. Encourage them to express their concerns or questions regarding screen time.

Collaborative Decision-Making

Involve your child in decisions about screen time rules and goals. Collaborative decision-making fosters a sense of ownership and responsibility.

Address Challenges Together

If challenges arise regarding screen time, address them together as a family. Problem-solving as a team reinforces the importance of cooperation and understanding.

Digital Detox Together

Consider implementing periodic digital detoxes as a family. Dedicate a day or weekend to unplugging from screens and enjoying offline activities.

Stay Informed

Stay informed about the latest trends and apps in the digital world. This knowledge allows you to guide your child effectively and address emerging challenges.

Supporting children in developing healthy digital habits involves setting realistic goals, encouraging alternative activities, and leading by example as parents. By fostering a balanced approach to screen time, parents can help their children navigate the digital landscape while promoting physical, emotional, and social well-being. Parental role modeling plays a crucial role in shaping a child's attitude towards technology and screens, making it essential for parents to demonstrate responsible and mindful screen time habits themselves.

8

RESOURCES AND TOOLS FOR PARENTS

PARENTAL RESOURCES FOR ADDRESSING SOCIAL MEDIA
ADDICTION

Parenting in the digital age comes with its unique set of challenges, one of which is addressing social media addiction among children and teenagers. The ever-evolving landscape of technology and social media platforms can be overwhelming for parents striving to strike a balance between allowing their children to benefit from the digital world and protecting them from its potential harms. In this chapter, we will explore the objective of providing practical tools and resources to support parents in addressing social media addiction in their households. We'll delve into the significance of seeking guidance and utilizing resources to navigate the challenges of parenting in the digital age effectively.

RECOMMENDED BOOKS AND WEBSITES ON PARENTING AND SOCIAL MEDIA

Importance of Expert Advice

Navigating the complex landscape of parenting in the digital age requires guidance and insights from experts in the field. Seeking advice and expertise in addressing social media addiction is of paramount importance for parents. This section will discuss the significance of expert advice and its role in shaping effective parenting strategies.

Understanding the Digital Age Challenge

The digital age has ushered in unprecedented challenges for parents. The landscape of technology and social media is constantly evolving, making it essential for parents to stay informed about the latest developments and their potential impact on children.

Expert advice provides parents with a deeper understanding of the challenges posed by social media addiction. These experts often conduct research, analyze trends, and offer practical solutions based on their findings.

Informed Decision-Making

Parents must make informed decisions about their child's screen time, online activities, and exposure to social media. Expert insights provide the knowledge necessary to make these decisions confidently.

Expert advice helps parents assess the potential risks and benefits associated with social media use, enabling them to create a balanced approach that supports their child's well-being.

Recognizing the Signs

Social media addiction may manifest in subtle ways that are not immediately apparent to parents. Experts can educate parents about the signs and symptoms of addiction, enabling earlier recognition and intervention.

Tailored Strategies

Every child is unique, and what works for one may not work for another. Experts can help parents tailor their strategies to their child's specific needs, taking into account factors such as age, personality, and interests.

Building Digital Literacy

Digital literacy is a crucial skill for children in the digital age. Experts can guide parents in fostering critical thinking, responsible online behavior, and digital literacy in their children.

Coping with Challenges

Parenting in the digital age can be challenging, and experts can offer coping strategies and support for parents facing difficulties related to social media addiction.

List of Recommended Books and Websites

To equip parents with valuable insights, tips, and strategies for navigating digital parenting and addressing social media addiction, we have curated a list of recommended books and websites. These resources provide a wealth of knowledge and guidance from experts in the field of parenting and technology. Let's explore some of these valuable sources:

Recommended Books

- "The Tech-Wise Family: Everyday Steps for Putting Technology in Its Proper Place" by Andy Crouch:

Author's Expertise

Andy Crouch is an author, speaker, and thought leader in the intersection of technology and faith. His book offers a comprehensive guide for families on how to cultivate healthy relationships with technology.

Key Takeaways

The book provides practical advice on setting boundaries, fostering face-to-face interactions, and nurturing a family culture that values meaningful connections over screen time.

- "iGen: Why Today's Super-Connected Kids Are

Growing Up Less Rebellious, More Tolerant, Less Happy – and Completely Unprepared for Adulthood" by Jean M. Twenge:

Author's Expertise

Jean M. Twenge is a psychologist and author known for her research on generational differences, particularly the iGen generation (born in the mid-1990s to mid-2000s). Her work sheds light on the impact of technology on this generation.

Key Takeaways

The book explores the trends and challenges faced by the iGen generation, offering insights into the role of technology, social media, and screen time in their lives.

- "The Digital Parenting Handbook: How to Know What Weird Apps Are on Your Kid's Phone" by Matt McKee: *Author's Expertise*

Matt McKee is a speaker, author, and digital strategist with expertise in helping parents navigate the digital landscape and understand their children's online activities.

Key Takeaways

This handbook provides parents with practical tools and advice for understanding and monitoring the apps and online platforms their children use.

- "Reset Your Child's Brain: A Four-Week Plan to End Meltdowns, Raise Grades, and Boost Social Skills by Reversing the Effects of Electronic Screen-Time" by Victoria L. Dunckley, MD:

Author's Expertise

Dr. Victoria L. Dunckley is an integrative child psychiatrist with extensive experience in treating children and adolescents impacted by excessive screen time.

Key Takeaways

The book offers a four-week plan to reset a child's brain by reducing screen time and promoting healthier digital habits. It explores the link between screen time and various behavioral and mental health challenges.

Recommended Websites

- Common Sense Media (commonsensemedia.org):

Expertise

Common Sense Media is a trusted source for parents seeking guidance on age-appropriate media content, including movies, TV shows, books, and apps. They provide comprehensive reviews and recommendations.

Key Features

Parents can access reviews, ratings, and educational resources to make informed decisions about what content is suitable for their children. The site also offers articles and tips on digital parenting.

- NetSmartz Workshop (netsmartz.org):

Expertise

NetSmartz Workshop is an initiative by the National Center for Missing & Exploited Children (NCMEC) to educate children and parents about online safety.

Key Features

The website offers resources, videos, and educational materials to teach children and parents about online safety, privacy, and responsible online behavior.

- Screenagers (screenagersmovie.com):

Expertise

"Screenagers" is a documentary film directed by Delaney Ruston, a physician and filmmaker. The film explores the impact of screen time on children's lives.

Key Features

The website provides resources, discussion guides, and information about the film, which can be a valuable tool for sparking conversations about screen time and digital habits within families and communities.

- Parenting for a Digital Future (blogs.lse.ac.uk/ parenting4digitalfuture):

Expertise

This blog is hosted by the London School of Economics and Political Science (LSE) and features articles and research findings related to parenting in the digital age.

Key Features

Parents can access academic research, expert opinions, and insights on a wide range of topics related to digital parenting, including screen time, online safety, and digital literacy.

In the digital age, seeking expert advice and incorporating expert insights into parenting strategies is crucial for addressing social media addiction and navigating the challenges of digital parenting. Recommended books and websites offer a wealth of knowledge and guidance from experts in the field of parenting and technology. These resources empower parents with the tools they need to make informed decisions, set appropriate boundaries, and foster responsible digital habits in their children. By leveraging the expertise provided by these sources, parents can create a healthier and more balanced digital environment for their families.

APPS AND TOOLS FOR MONITORING AND MANAGING SCREEN TIME

Range of Available Tools

As parents navigate the challenges of raising children in the digital age, an array of apps and tools have emerged to assist them in monitoring and managing their children's screen time effectively. In this section, we will explore the various apps and tools available to parents for this purpose and discuss the benefits they offer in terms of setting limits, tracking app usage, and enforcing screen-free periods.

The Digital Age Parenting Challenge

Parenting in the digital age brings unique challenges, including concerns about excessive screen time and its impact on children's physical and mental health. As children increasingly engage with digital devices, parents seek ways to strike a balance between technology use and other important aspects of their children's lives.

Importance of Monitoring and Managing Screen Time

Monitoring and managing screen time are essential components of responsible digital parenting. These practices empower parents to:

Set healthy boundaries

Parents can establish appropriate limits on screen time to ensure that their children have time for other activities, such as homework, physical exercise, and face-to-face interactions.

Ensure age-appropriate content

Parents can monitor the content their children access to ensure it is suitable for their age and maturity level.

Promote digital literacy

By tracking their children's app usage, parents can encourage discussions about responsible online behavior and digital literacy.

Address addiction and dependency

Monitoring screen time helps parents identify signs of addiction or dependency on digital devices and take proactive steps to address these issues.

Benefits of Screen Time Management Tools

Screen time management tools offer several benefits to parents:

Transparency

Parents gain insight into their children's digital activities, allowing them to make informed decisions about screen time limits.

Customization

Many tools allow parents to set individualized screen time limits for each child based on their age, needs, and responsibilities.

App control

Parents can monitor and manage the apps their children use, ensuring they have access to age-appropriate and safe content.

App usage tracking

Tools often provide detailed reports on app usage, helping parents identify potential concerns or addictive behaviors.

Screen-free periods

Parents can schedule screen-free periods to encourage offline activities, family time, and restful sleep.

Examples of Parental Control Apps

Parental control apps are a valuable resource for parents seeking to monitor and manage their children's screen time effectively. These apps offer a range of features designed to promote responsible technology use and ensure a healthy balance between digital and offline activities. Here are some examples of parental control apps and how they contribute to effective screen time management:

- **Qustodio**

Key Features:

Screen Time Monitoring

Qustodio allows parents to track their child's screen time across various devices, providing insights into daily, weekly, and monthly usage.

App and Website Blocking

Parents can block access to specific apps and websites that they deem inappropriate or distracting.

App Usage Reports

The app provides detailed reports on the apps and games their child uses, helping parents identify potential concerns.

Time Limits

Parents can set daily or weekly screen time limits, helping children manage their device usage effectively.

- **Bark**

Key Features:

Content Monitoring

Bark uses advanced algorithms to monitor text messages, emails, and social media platforms for signs of cyberbullying, self-harm, or inappropriate content.

Screen Time Scheduling

Parents can schedule screen-free periods, ensuring that children have designated times for other activities.

Alerts and Notifications

Bark sends alerts to parents if it detects potentially concerning online activity, allowing for timely intervention.

App Blocking

Parents can block access to specific apps or games to promote focused and responsible screen time.

- **Screen Time**

  Key Features:

Daily Time Limits

Screen Time allows parents to set daily screen time limits for each device, helping children manage their usage.

Bedtime Mode

Parents can schedule bedtime mode to ensure that screens are turned off during designated hours to promote restful sleep.

App Monitoring

The app provides insights into the apps used most frequently, allowing parents to identify potential areas for adjustment.

Content Filters

Screen Time offers content filtering to block access to inappropriate websites and content.

Built-In Tools in Operating Systems

In addition to third-party parental control apps, many operating systems offer built-in tools that enable parents to monitor and manage screen time effectively. Let's explore some of these built-in tools and how they can be utilized for screen time regulation:

- **Apple's Screen Time**

Key Features:

App Limits

Parents can set daily or weekly time limits for specific app categories or individual apps.

Downtime

Downtime allows parents to schedule periods when only essential apps and phone calls are accessible, promoting family time and rest.

Content and Privacy Restrictions

Parents can restrict access to certain content and privacy settings, ensuring age-appropriate usage.

Usage Reports

Screen Time provides weekly reports on screen time usage and app activity.

- **Google's Digital Wellbeing**

Key Features:

Dashboard

Google's Digital Wellbeing dashboard offers insights into screen time, app usage, and notifications.

App Timers

Parents can set daily time limits for specific apps to encourage responsible usage.

Wind Down

Wind Down mode helps create a bedtime routine by reducing screen brightness and enabling grayscale mode during designated hours.

Focus Mode

Focus mode allows users to temporarily pause distracting apps.

- **Microsoft Family Safety**

Key Features:

Screen Time Limits

Parents can set screen time limits for Windows devices, Xbox consoles, and Android devices.

App and Game Filters

Parents can restrict access to age-inappropriate apps and games.

Activity Reporting

Microsoft Family Safety provides activity reports, including screen time usage, app activity, and web browsing history.

As parents seek to address the challenges of parenting in the digital age, a range of apps and tools are available to assist them in monitoring and managing their children's screen time effectively. These tools empower parents to set limits, track app usage, and enforce screen-free periods, ultimately promoting a healthier balance between technology use and other essential aspects of their children's lives. Whether through dedicated parental control apps or built-in tools within operating systems, parents have access to resources that support responsible digital parenting and help foster a more balanced and mindful approach to screen time.

LOCAL SUPPORT GROUPS AND COUNSELING SERVICES

Importance of Local Support

In the journey to address social media addiction within families, the significance of seeking support from local communities and professional counseling services cannot be overstated. This section delves into the importance of local support and highlights the benefits of local support groups and counseling services in addressing social media addiction effectively.

The Value of Local Support

Parenting can be an isolating experience, particularly when faced with complex challenges like social media addiction. Seeking support from local communities and professional services provides several advantages:

Understanding and Empathy

Local support groups and counselors can offer empathy and understanding, as they are familiar with the unique challenges parents and children face in the digital age.

Shared Experiences

Parents in local support groups often share similar experiences and challenges. This common ground fosters a sense of community and mutual support.

Local Resources

Local communities offer access to resources and services tailored to the specific needs of the community, including counseling services and workshops.

Benefits of Local Support Groups

Local support groups play a vital role in helping parents address social media addiction within their families. Let's explore the benefits they offer:

Joining Local Support Groups

Sharing Experiences

Local support groups provide a safe space for parents to share their experiences, challenges, and successes related to social media addiction. This sharing fosters a sense of belonging and reduces the isolation often felt by parents facing these issues.

Learning from Others

Hearing about the strategies and solutions other parents have found effective can be invaluable. Parents in support groups often offer practical advice and tips based on their own experiences.

Emotional Support

Dealing with social media addiction can be emotionally taxing. Local support groups offer emotional support and a sense of camaraderie, helping parents cope with the stress and uncertainty of the journey.

Accountability

Being part of a group can provide parents with a sense of accountability. Sharing progress and setbacks with others can motivate parents to stay committed to addressing social media addiction within their families.

Networking

Local support groups can connect parents with resources and professionals in the community who specialize in addressing addiction and mental health issues.

Role of Professional Counseling Services

Expert Guidance

Professional counseling services play a crucial role in providing expert guidance and intervention for families dealing with social media addiction. Here are some key points to consider:

Individualized Support

Professional counselors can assess each family's unique situation and provide individualized support tailored to their needs.

Family Dynamics

Counselors are trained to understand and address the complex dynamics that arise within families dealing with addiction. They can help families navigate these challenges effectively.

Therapeutic Techniques

Counselors employ therapeutic techniques that can help both parents and children develop healthier coping strategies and communication skills.

Coordinated Care

In cases where social media addiction is linked to underlying mental health issues, counselors can coordinate care with other healthcare professionals to ensure comprehensive treatment.

Confidentiality

Professional counseling services offer a confidential and non-judgmental space for families to discuss their concerns, ensuring privacy and trust.

Potential Benefits of Professional Help

Seeking professional help can yield several benefits for families addressing social media addiction:

Early Intervention

Professional counselors can identify signs of addiction and intervene early, mitigating the long-term impact of excessive social media use.

Communication Improvement

Counseling can improve family communication by teaching parents and children effective communication skills, fostering understanding, and reducing conflicts.

Behavioral Modification

Counselors use evidence-based techniques to address addiction-related behaviors, helping children and parents modify their behaviors for healthier outcomes.

Relapse Prevention

Professional counseling services equip families with strategies to prevent relapse and maintain the progress made in addressing addiction.

Holistic Approach

Counselors take a holistic approach, addressing not only addiction but also underlying emotional, psychological, and relational factors that contribute to the issue.

In the journey to address social media addiction within families, local support groups and professional counseling services play pivotal roles. The importance of seeking support from local communities and professionals cannot be understated. These resources offer understanding, empathy, shared experiences, and expert guidance that can significantly enhance a family's ability to address addiction effectively.

Local support groups provide parents with a sense of community, opportunities to learn from others, emotional support, and accountability. They create a network of parents who share similar challenges and can offer practical advice and resources.

Professional counseling services bring a wealth of expertise, including individualized support, an understanding of family dynamics, therapeutic techniques, and a confidential space for families to address addiction and related issues. Seeking professional help can lead to early intervention, improved communication, behavioral modification, relapse prevention, and a holistic approach to addressing addiction.

By combining the strengths of local support groups and professional counseling services, parents can create a robust support system that empowers them to address social media addiction and promote healthier family dynamics. These resources contribute to a comprehensive approach that prioritizes the well-being of children and families in the digital age.

9
CASE STUDIES: REALLIFE EXPERIENCES

In the digital age, the challenges of parenting have taken on new dimensions, and one of the most pressing issues is social media addiction. While we've discussed strategies, resources, and professional guidance in previous chapters, real-life stories offer a unique perspective that can resonate deeply with parents. These stories provide a window into the lives of individuals who have faced social media addiction head-on, offering valuable lessons and inspiration to others on a similar journey.

PARENT TESTIMONIALS AND INTERVIEWS

Firsthand Accounts of Challenges

In Chapter 9 of our book, we explore the real-life challenges faced by parents due to social media addiction within their families through firsthand accounts in the form of parent testimonials and interviews. These accounts provide valuable insights into the diverse range of challenges experienced by parents in the digital age.

The Power of Parent Testimonials

Parent testimonials and interviews are powerful tools for conveying the real-world experiences of those who have grappled with social media addiction within their families. By sharing their stories, these parents shed light on the complex and often emotional challenges they faced.

These firsthand accounts offer authenticity and relatability, helping other parents who may be navigating similar issues feel understood and less alone in their struggles.

Showcase of Diversity

The parent testimonials and interviews featured in this section will showcase the diversity of challenges related to social media addiction. We will include accounts from parents who have faced various aspects of the issue, such as excessive screen time, online bullying, social isolation, and academic impacts.

By highlighting a wide range of challenges, we aim to provide a comprehensive perspective on the multifaceted nature of social media addiction and its effects on parent-child relationships.

Impact on Relationships

Emotional and Relational Aspects

Within the parent testimonials and interviews, we will delve into the specific ways in which social media addiction has impacted parent-child relationships. These impacts encompass emotional, relational, and psychological dimensions.

Some of the key areas of impact that will be explored include:

- Communication breakdowns
- Increased conflict and tension
- Emotional distancing
- Reduced quality time together
- Erosion of trust
- Academic and behavioral changes in children

Through these accounts, readers will gain a deep understanding of the toll that social media addiction can take on family dynamics.

Personal Narratives

Personal narratives will be featured to provide a window into the emotions and experiences of parents. These narratives will not only describe the challenges faced but also convey the emotional journey of parents as they grappled with their child's addiction and sought solutions.

These personal narratives will offer a humanizing perspective, allowing readers to connect with the emotional turmoil and resilience of parents in the face of adversity.

Strategies Implemented

Diverse Approaches

The parent testimonials and interviews will not only highlight the challenges but also showcase the various strategies employed by parents to address social media addiction within their families.

These strategies will encompass a wide spectrum, including:

- Setting boundaries and screen time limits
- Seeking professional help and counseling
- Implementing digital detoxes
- Fostering open communication
- Engaging in shared activities and hobbies
- Leveraging parental control apps and tools

By presenting diverse approaches, readers will gain insights into the multifaceted nature of solutions available to address social media addiction.

Lessons Learned

Each parent testimonial and interview will conclude with reflections on the lessons learned throughout their journey.

These insights may include:

- The importance of early intervention
- The value of open and non-judgmental communication
- The need for empathy and understanding
- The role of professional guidance
- The significance of family bonding and shared experiences

These lessons learned will provide actionable takeaways for other parents facing similar challenges.

Parent testimonials and interviews within Chapter 9 will offer a rich and multifaceted exploration of the challenges, impact on relationships, and strategies employed by parents in response to social media addiction within their families. These firsthand accounts will provide readers with relatable stories, emotional depth, and practical insights, enhancing their understanding of the complexities of parenting in the digital age. By sharing these personal journeys, we aim to inspire and empower parents to navigate their own challenges with resilience and hope.

LESSONS LEARNED AND SUCCESSFUL STRATEGIES

Insights from Successful Cases

In Chapter 9 of our book, we delve into the valuable insights gained from parents who successfully addressed social media addiction within their households. These success stories offer profound lessons that shed light on the positive outcomes achieved and the strategies employed to mitigate the impact of social media addiction.

Lessons Learned from Successful Cases

Successful cases provide a treasure trove of insights for parents grappling with social media addiction challenges. These lessons encapsulate various facets of parenting in the digital age and underscore essential takeaways:

Early Recognition and Intervention

One recurring theme in successful cases is the importance of early recognition and intervention. Parents who spotted the signs of addiction in their children at an early stage were better equipped to address the issue effectively. They emphasized the significance of staying vigilant and attuned to behavioral changes that might indicate addiction.

Persistence and Consistency

Another critical lesson from successful cases is the value of persistence and consistency in implementing strategies. Overcoming social media addiction often requires time and effort. Parents who remained steadfast in their approach, even in the face of resistance, saw more significant improvements over time.

Adaptability and Flexibility

Successful parents recognized the need for adaptability and flexibility in addressing evolving challenges. They understood that what worked initially might need adjustments as circumstances changed. This adaptability allowed them to tailor their strategies to their child's specific needs and circumstances.

Empathy and Understanding

The role of empathy and understanding in parent-child relationships emerged as a prominent theme. Parents who approached the issue with empathy, refraining from judgment, and actively listening to their child's perspective, found that their children were more receptive to guidance and support.

Parental Role Modeling

Parents who successfully addressed social media addiction recognized the profound impact of parental role modeling. By demonstrating responsible technology use and setting a positive example, these parents encouraged their children to adopt healthier digital habits.

Acknowledgment of Complexity

Successful cases underscored the recognition of addiction as a complex issue encompassing both digital and emotional components. Parents understood that addressing social media addiction required a multifaceted approach, addressing not only screen time but also underlying emotional needs and coping mechanisms.

Setting Boundaries

Effective Boundary Setting

Within successful cases, we can explore in-depth how parents set and enforced boundaries to mitigate the impact of social media addiction. This section provides practical insights into creating effective rules and guidelines that contribute to successful outcomes.

Defining Clear and Age-Appropriate Screen Time Limits

Successful parents emphasized the importance of defining clear and age-appropriate screen time limits. These limits were established based on the child's age, developmental stage, and individual needs. By setting these boundaries, parents provided structure and guidance for healthy technology use.

Involving Children in Rule-Making

Parents who achieved success actively involved their children in the rule-making process. This inclusion promoted a sense of ownership and understanding. Children were more likely to adhere to boundaries they had a hand in creating, leading to more cooperative and effective enforcement.

Utilizing Parental Control Apps and Tools

Some successful cases highlighted the use of parental control apps and tools to enforce boundaries. These technologies allowed parents to monitor and manage their child's screen time, ensuring that limits were adhered to. Parental control apps were seen as valuable tools in the digital parenting toolkit.

Addressing Resistance and Negotiating Compromises

Successful parents also addressed resistance and learned effective strategies for negotiating compromises with their children. They recognized that resistance was a natural response to change and adopted approaches that fostered cooperation rather than confrontation.

Improving Communication

Role of Improved Communication

Successful cases often underscored the role of improved communication in achieving positive outcomes. This section discusses how enhanced communication strategies positively influenced parent-child relationships and contributed to overcoming social media addiction.

Creating a Safe and Non-Judgmental Environment

Successful parents emphasized the importance of creating a safe and non-judgmental environment for their children to express themselves. They ensured that their children felt comfortable sharing their thoughts, concerns, and experiences related to social media without fear of punishment or criticism.

Actively Listening to Children's Concerns

Improved communication involved actively listening to children's concerns and perspectives. Successful parents practiced active listening, which included maintaining eye contact, paraphrasing, and showing empathy. This approach allowed parents to better understand their children's viewpoints and emotional experiences.

Using Open-Ended Questions and Paraphrasing

Effective communication strategies included the use of open-ended questions and paraphrasing. These techniques encouraged children to express themselves more openly and facilitated deeper conversations. Paraphrasing ensured that parents accurately understood their child's thoughts and feelings. *Encouraging Children to Share Experiences*

Successful parents actively encouraged their children to share their experiences and challenges related to social media. By fostering open and ongoing dialogues, parents were better equipped to identify issues early and provide timely support.

Seeking Professional Help

The Importance of Professional Intervention

Successful cases highlighted the importance of seeking professional help as a successful strategy in addressing social media addiction. This section provides examples of how professional intervention positively contributed to overcoming addiction within families.

The Role of Therapists and Counselors

Parents who achieved success recognized the instrumental role of therapists and counselors. These professionals played a crucial part in assessing and addressing addiction-related behaviors. They employed evidence-based therapeutic techniques to help children and parents develop healthier coping strategies and communication skills.

Benefits of Individualized Support

Professional counselors offered individualized support tailored to the unique needs of each family. They conducted thorough assessments to understand the specific challenges and dynamics at play. This personalized approach allowed for targeted interventions that addressed the root causes of addiction.

Coordination of Care with Other Professionals

In cases where social media addiction was linked to underlying mental health issues, successful parents highlighted the importance of coordinating care with other healthcare professionals.

This collaboration ensured comprehensive treatment that addressed both the addiction and the underlying emotional or psychological factors.

Creating a Confidential and Non-Judgmental Space

Seeking professional help provided families with a confidential and non-judgmental space to address addiction. This safe environment allowed children to express themselves openly and honestly, facilitating the therapeutic process.

Successful cases offer a wealth of insights into addressing social media addiction. These stories illuminate the lessons learned, effective boundary-setting strategies, improved communication techniques, and the importance of seeking professional intervention. By exploring these successful approaches, parents can better navigate the challenges of social media addiction and cultivate healthier relationships in the digital age.

OVERCOMING OBSTACLES AND CELEBRATING VICTORIES

Exploration of Obstacles

The Multifaceted Nature of Obstacles

Addressing social media addiction within a family context is no simple task. Parents often encounter a multifaceted array of obstacles that test their resolve and patience. These obstacles include:

Resistance and Pushback

Many parents grapple with resistance and pushback from their children when attempting to establish healthier screen time boundaries. This resistance can manifest as defiance, emotional outbursts, or even withdrawal.

Emotional Distress

Social media addiction often takes a toll on the emotional well-being of both children and parents. Families may experience heightened stress, anxiety, and conflicts as they confront the addiction's impact.

Academic and Behavioral Repercussions

Addiction can lead to a decline in academic performance and behavioral issues in children. Parents must navigate the educational challenges posed by excessive screen time.

Peer Pressure and External Influences

Peer pressure and the influence of online communities can exacerbate addiction. Parents face the challenge of helping their children resist negative online peer pressure.

Pervasive Nature of Social Media

In the digital age, social media's ubiquity poses a constant challenge. Children have easy access to social platforms, making it challenging for parents to monitor and regulate their online activities.

The Resilience of Parents:

What emerges as a common thread among parents facing these obstacles is their remarkable resilience. Despite the myriad challenges, parents remain steadfast in their commitment to their children's well-being and the overall health of their family dynamics.

Parents navigate emotional turmoil, engage in difficult conversations, and tirelessly seek solutions. Their determination serves as a beacon of hope for others facing similar hurdles.

Creative Solutions

Innovative Approaches to Overcoming Obstacles

An inspiring aspect of the journey to address social media addiction is the innovative solutions parents craft to surmount specific obstacles. This section highlights the creativity and resourcefulness that parents in the digital age demonstrate.

Unique and Effective Strategies

Parents have devised unique and effective approaches to address social media addiction. Some examples of these innovative solutions include:

Transforming Screen Time

Some parents have transformed screen time into opportunities for learning and expression. They have encouraged their children to engage with educational content, creative apps, and online communities that foster positive growth.

Leveraging Technology for Connection

Forward-thinking parents have leveraged technology to foster family connections. They have discovered shared apps, interactive games, and virtual experiences that bring family members closer despite the digital distractions.

Collaborating with Schools

Recognizing the need for a comprehensive approach, some parents have collaborated with schools to establish digital well-being programs. These programs educate students about responsible technology use and equip them with the skills needed to navigate the digital landscape safely.

Offline Events and Activities

Parents have organized offline events and activities to counterbalance excessive screen time. These include family outings, nature excursions, and hobbies that encourage physical activity and face-to-face interactions.

Support Groups and Mentorship

Encouraging children to participate in support groups and mentorship programs has proven effective. These initiatives provide children with a sense of community and guidance from peers and mentors who have overcome similar challenges.

These creative solutions not only address immediate obstacles but also contribute to long-term digital well-being and the promotion of harmonious family dynamics.

Celebrating Victories

Positive Outcomes and Victories

Throughout the parenting journey, there are moments of celebration and victories that parents can look back on with pride and joy. These positive outcomes result from their unwavering dedication to addressing social media addiction.

Victories span a wide range of areas, including:

Improved Parent-Child Relationships

Parents have reported significant improvements in parent-child relationships. Trust and open communication are reestablished, fostering a deeper bond between parents and their children.

Reduction in Screen Time

Efforts to reduce screen time have often yielded positive results, with children developing healthier technology habits. This reduction in screen time has been associated with improved well-being and academic performance.

Empowerment of Children

Parents have empowered their children to make informed and responsible digital choices. Through open dialogue and guidance, children have gained the skills necessary to navigate the digital landscape safely and responsibly.

A Sense of Accomplishment

Parents have expressed a sense of accomplishment and fulfillment as they witnessed positive changes within their families. These changes reaffirm the importance of their efforts and inspire them to continue promoting digital well-being.

The Ripple Effect

Celebrating victories goes beyond personal achievements; it involves recognizing the broader impact on family dynamics and relationships. Parents who successfully navigated social media addiction often observed a ripple effect of positive changes that extended beyond their immediate family unit:

Siblings Benefit

Improved family dynamics and shared activities often benefit siblings, creating a more harmonious and supportive sibling relationship.

Extended Family and Friends

Extended family members and friends frequently notice positive shifts in the child's behavior and well-being. This creates a supportive network that reinforces the positive changes initiated by parents.

Schools and Communities

Schools and communities benefit from parents' advocacy for responsible technology use. Parents often engage with schools to promote digital literacy and well-being programs, contributing to a safer and more informed digital environment for all children.

By discussing the multifaceted obstacles encountered, the innovative solutions devised, and the positive outcomes achieved, this section provides readers with a comprehensive understanding of the challenges and triumphs of addressing social media addiction. It serves as a source of inspiration and practical guidance for parents navigating similar journeys, fostering hope and empowerment in their efforts to promote digital well-being and family harmony.

INTEGRATION AND APPLICATION OF LESSONS

Practical Advice Based on Experiences

Insights into Practical Solutions

The experiences shared by parents in Chapter 9 provide a rich source of practical advice for readers. These insights encompass a wide range of strategies and approaches that have proven effective in addressing social media addiction within families.

Setting and Enforcing Boundaries

Many parents shared their experiences of setting clear and consistent boundaries regarding screen time and social media use. These boundaries often included age-appropriate limits and guidelines for responsible digital behavior. Readers can draw from these experiences to establish their own effective boundaries.

Open Communication

Successful cases frequently emphasized the importance of open and honest communication between parents and children. Parents shared techniques for creating a safe space for conversations about social media use, fostering understanding and cooperation. Readers can learn from these communication strategies.

Alternative Activities

Parents often introduced alternative activities and hobbies to divert their children's attention from excessive screen time. These activities ranged from outdoor sports to creative arts and helped children develop diverse interests. Readers can gain inspiration for similar activities.

Professional Support

Several parents highlighted the pivotal role of professional intervention, such as therapy and counseling, in addressing addiction. These experiences underscore the importance of seeking professional help when necessary. Readers can recognize the signs that may warrant professional support.

Tech-Free Zones

The establishment of tech-free zones and designated device-free times in the home was a common approach. Parents found that these zones promoted face-to-face interaction and quality bonding time. Readers can consider implementing similar tech-free zones in their households.

Tailoring Solutions to Specific Situations

The experiences shared in Chapter 9 demonstrate that there is no one-size-fits-all solution to addressing social media addiction.

Instead, parents tailored their approaches to the specific needs and dynamics of their families.

Assessing Family Dynamics

Readers can glean insights into the importance of assessing their own family dynamics and understanding the unique challenges posed by social media addiction.

Recognizing Individual Needs

Successful parents often recognized the individual needs of their children and adjusted their strategies accordingly. Readers can learn to identify the specific needs of their own children.

Flexibility and Adaptation

Flexibility and adaptation were key themes in many experiences. Readers can appreciate the need to adapt their strategies as their children grow and their digital habits evolve.

Relatability and Empowerment

The Relatability of Shared Experiences

One of the strengths of Chapter 9 lies in its ability to convey the relatability of shared experiences. Readers can connect with these stories on a personal level, recognizing their own challenges and struggles within the narratives of others. The relatability of these experiences serves as a source of comfort and validation for readers who may have felt alone in their journey.

Validation of Parenting Struggles

Readers may find solace in realizing that they are not alone in their parenting struggles. The challenges faced by the parents in these stories resonate with the difficulties many readers encounter in their efforts to manage their children's screen time and social media use.

Understanding the Impact

Readers can gain a deeper understanding of the impact of social media addiction on family dynamics, academic performance, and emotional well-being. This understanding can help them contextualize their own experiences.

Empowerment through Success Stories

The success stories shared in Chapter 9 are a powerful source of empowerment for readers. These stories demonstrate that positive change is achievable and that dedicated efforts can lead to meaningful improvements in family life.

Inspiration for Change

Readers can draw inspiration from the journeys of parents who successfully addressed social media addiction. These stories provide hope and motivation for readers who may be facing similar challenges.

Belief in Positive Outcomes

Through these success stories, readers can develop a belief in the possibility of positive outcomes. They can see that with commitment and the right strategies, it is possible to overcome social media addiction and build healthier family relationships.

Rekindling Hope

For readers who may have felt discouraged or overwhelmed, these stories can rekindle hope and optimism. They serve as a reminder that change is within reach.

10

THE ROAD AHEAD: SUSTAINING CHANGE

As parents, we understand that the journey of managing social media usage within our families is an ongoing one. The changes we've implemented and the lessons we've learned throughout this book have set the stage for a brighter and more balanced future, but the road ahead requires our continued commitment and vigilance.

MAKING SOCIAL MEDIA A HEALTHY AND BALANCED PART OF FAMILY LIFE

Integration Strategies

Understanding the Role of Social Media

To effectively integrate social media into family life, it is essential to first understand its role in the modern world. Social media has become a pervasive aspect of society, impacting how we communicate, access information, and entertain ourselves. Recognizing its significance is the foundation for responsible integration.

Impact on Family Dynamics

Discuss how social media affects family dynamics. It can facilitate communication, but it can also be a source of distraction and conflict. Understanding these dynamics helps in setting integration goals.

Setting Reasonable Limits and Boundaries

One of the fundamental strategies for achieving a healthy balance is the establishment of reasonable limits and boundaries. These boundaries serve as guidelines to prevent social media from overshadowing other critical aspects of family life.

Defining Screen-Free Zones

Discuss the concept of creating specific areas or times in the home as screen-free zones. These areas, such as the dining table or bedrooms, are reserved for face-to-face interactions and family bonding.

Tech-Free Times

Emphasize the importance of tech-free times during the day, such as during family meals or before bedtime. This ensures that family members are fully present and engaged with each other.

Age-Appropriate Guidelines

Tailoring social media rules to the age and maturity of each family member. Younger children may have stricter limits, while older teenagers may have more autonomy, accompanied by responsible usage guidelines.

Consistency

Enforce these boundaries consistently, modeling the behavior you expect from your children. This consistency helps establish the expectation that family time is precious and uninterrupted by screens.

Balancing Screen Time

Achieving a balanced integration of social media into family life involves managing screen time effectively. This includes:

Screen Time Tracking

Utilizing screen time tracking apps and features provided by devices to monitor and assess individual and family screen time. This data can inform discussions and adjustments to screen time limits.

Quality Over Quantity

Emphasize the importance of the quality of screen time over quantity. Encourage children to engage in meaningful and educational content rather than mindless scrolling.

Tech-Free Activities

Promoting a variety of tech-free activities that family members can enjoy together. These activities foster connection and serve as alternatives to excessive screen time.

Promoting Digital Well-being and Mindfulness

Understanding Digital Well-being

Digital well-being refers to having a healthy and balanced relationship with technology, including social media.

To promote digital well-being within the family:

Educate Family Members

Help family members understand the concept of digital well-being and its importance for mental and emotional health.

Identify Warning Signs

Teach children to recognize warning signs of excessive social media use, such as irritability, sleep disturbances, or declining academic performance.

Encourage Self-Reflection

Promote self-reflection on the impact of social media use. Encourage family members to assess how their online interactions affect their overall well-being.

Practical Tips for Mindful Social Media Use

Mindful social media use involves engaging with digital platforms with intention and awareness. Here are practical tips to foster mindfulness:

Set Daily Intentions

Encourage family members to set intentions for their social media use each day. Are they using it for connection, entertainment, or information?

Practice Digital Detoxes

Periodically, engage in digital detoxes as a family. This involves taking breaks from social media to reconnect with offline activities and each other.

Mindful Posting

Teach the importance of thinking before posting. Encourage children to consider the potential impact of their online content on themselves and others.

Limit Notifications

Limit the frequency of notifications to reduce distractions and promote focused, intentional use of social media.

Open Communication

Foster open communication within the family about social media experiences. Encourage children to share their online encounters and feelings, especially if they encounter cyberbullying or negative content.

Model Mindful Behavior

As parents, model mindful social media use. Children often emulate the behavior they observe, so demonstrating a healthy relationship with technology sets a positive example.

Striking a Balance

Making social media a healthy and balanced part of family life involves a thoughtful integration of technology, setting reasonable limits and boundaries, and promoting digital well-being and mindfulness. By recognizing the role of social media in modern life and establishing guidelines that prioritize quality family time, parents can guide their children toward responsible and mindful social media usage. This approach fosters stronger family connections and equips children with the skills needed to navigate the digital world with wisdom and balance. The key is to strike a harmonious equilibrium where social media enhances family life rather than detracting from it.

REINFORCING POSITIVE HABITS AND BOUNDARIES

In this comprehensive exploration, we will delve into the critical aspects of reinforcing positive habits and boundaries in the context of social media use within families. Consistency, parental role-modeling, and practical techniques will be discussed in detail to provide a comprehensive understanding of these essential elements.

Consistency in Reinforcement

The Importance of Consistency

Consistency in reinforcing positive habits and boundaries is fundamental to their long-term effectiveness. Inconsistent enforcement can lead to confusion and undermine the established rules. Here, we will discuss why consistency matters and how it can be achieved.

Creating Predictability

Explain how consistent rules and consequences create predictability for children. When they know what to expect, they are more likely to adhere to the rules.

Avoiding Confusion

Discuss how inconsistent enforcement can lead to confusion and frustration among children. It can also create opportunities for negotiation and rule-bending.

Practical Techniques for Parents

Achieving consistency requires practical techniques that parents can implement. Here, we will explore these techniques in depth, including:

Clear Communication

The importance of clear communication regarding rules and expectations. Discuss techniques for explaining the reasons behind rules to children and how this fosters understanding.

Positive Reinforcement

The role of positive reinforcement in encouraging adherence to rules. Explore strategies such as praise and rewards for compliance with established boundaries.

Consequences

The use of consequences for rule violations. Discuss the importance of consequences being fair, reasonable, and directly related to the rule that was broken.

Consistent Enforcement

The need for parents to be consistent in enforcing consequences. Explain how wavering on consequences can lead to confusion and a weakening of boundaries.

Parental Role-Modeling

Highlighting Parental Role-Modeling

Parental role-modeling is a powerful tool in reinforcing positive habits and boundaries related to social media use. Children often learn by observing their parents, so setting a good example is crucial. In this section, we will emphasize the significance of parental role-modeling.

Lead by Example

Discuss how parents can lead by example by practicing healthy social media habits themselves. Explain that children are more likely to follow rules when they see their parents doing the same.

Openness to Learning

Emphasize that parents can also model the behavior of being open to learning and adapting to new technologies. This shows children that responsible technology use is an ongoing process.

Balancing Screen Time

Discuss the importance of parents demonstrating a balanced approach to screen time. This includes setting boundaries for their own social media use and prioritizing family time.

Practical Insights into Parental Role-Modeling

To effectively role-model positive behavior, parents need practical insights and strategies. This section will provide detailed guidance on how parents can become effective role models.

Setting Personal Boundaries

Discuss how parents can establish their own boundaries for social media use. This can include designating tech-free times and zones for themselves.

Engaging in Tech-Free Activities

Encourage parents to engage in tech-free activities with their children. Share ideas for quality bonding time that doesn't involve screens.

Open Communication

Explain how open communication about social media experiences can be part of parental role-modeling. Encourage parents to share their own challenges and successes in navigating the digital world.

Nurturing a Culture of Responsibility

Reinforcing positive habits and boundaries around social media use within the family is a multifaceted process that involves consistency in enforcement and effective parental rolemodeling. Consistency provides predictability and clarity, while parental role-modeling sets the tone for responsible technology use. Together, these elements nurture a culture of responsibility, where children learn to navigate the digital world with awareness, balance, and respect for established boundaries. Parents play a pivotal role in shaping their children's digital habits and ensuring that they grow into responsible and mindful users of technology.

CONTINUING TO PRIORITIZE MEANINGFUL CONNECTIONS

Ongoing Need for Prioritization

The Persistence of Meaningful Connections

In today's digital age, where screens and devices often dominate our lives, the enduring need for meaningful connections within families remains undiminished. Despite the allure and convenience of technology, the core of family bonds and relationships remains rooted in human connection. It's important to convey that while technology can facilitate communication and offer opportunities for connection, it should not replace or overshadow the essence of genuine human interactions.

Fulfillment and Well-being

Meaningful connections within the family are not just emotionally fulfilling; they are also integral to the overall wellbeing of both parents and children. Research has consistently shown that strong family bonds contribute to mental and emotional health. Children who feel connected to their families tend to have higher self-esteem, improved emotional regulation, and better overall mental health. Parents, too, experience greater life satisfaction and emotional support when they maintain meaningful connections with their children.

Strengthening Resilience

One of the lesser-discussed benefits of strong family relationships is their role in helping children build resilience. In the face of the challenges posed by the digital age, where cyberbullying, online peer pressure, and exposure to inappropriate content are prevalent, children need a solid support system. Healthy relationships within the family provide a safe haven where children can seek guidance, express their concerns, and find emotional support. This resilience, developed through strong family bonds, equips children to navigate the digital world with confidence and self-assuredness.

Quality vs. Quantity

It's essential to emphasize that the quality of time spent together is more important than the quantity. In today's busy world, where parents often juggle work, household responsibilities, and other commitments, finding extended periods of undistracted time can be challenging. However, it's the quality of interactions during the time available that truly matters. Parents can make the most of shorter, focused moments by engaging in meaningful conversations, active listening, and bonding activities.

Fostering Strong Relationships

Fostering strong relationships within families is an ongoing process that requires intentionality and effort. It involves a combination of quality time activities, the creation of family traditions, active participation in children's interests, and effective communication skills.

Quality Time Activities

Quality time activities are essential for strengthening bonds within the family. These activities are characterized by undivided attention, genuine engagement, and shared enjoyment. Family dinners, game nights, outdoor adventures, and shared hobbies are examples of quality time activities that promote togetherness. They create opportunities for laughter, connection, and memorable experiences that contribute to a sense of unity.

Creating Traditions

Family traditions hold a special place in the hearts of children and parents alike. These rituals, whether simple or elaborate, create a sense of continuity and belonging. They can be as straightforward as a weekly movie night, a monthly hiking excursion, or an annual holiday tradition. The key is consistency, as traditions build a shared history and reinforce the idea that family time is a valued and cherished part of life.

Active Participation

Active participation in children's interests and passions is a powerful way to foster strong relationships. It communicates to children that their pursuits are important and worthy of attention. Whether it's attending their soccer games, participating in their artistic endeavors, or exploring their hobbies, parents who actively engage in their children's activities create lasting memories and deep connections.

Communication Skills

Effective communication skills are the foundation of strong relationships within families. Parents can enhance their communication skills by practicing active listening, empathy, and creating a safe space for open dialogue. Active listening involves giving full attention, paraphrasing, and asking openended questions. Empathy allows parents to understand their children's perspectives, validate their feelings, and respond with compassion. Creating a safe space for open dialogue encourages children to express themselves freely, knowing that their thoughts and emotions will be respected and valued.

Open and Honest Conversations

The Significance of Openness

Open and honest conversations about the impact of social media on relationships are not only significant but also necessary in today's digital landscape. These conversations serve multiple purposes, including raising awareness, promoting understanding, resolving conflicts, and building trust.

Awareness and Understanding

Open conversations about the influence of social media raise awareness and foster a deeper understanding of its potential pitfalls. By discussing issues like cyberbullying, excessive screen time, and the impact of online relationships, parents can equip their children with the knowledge and tools to navigate the digital world safely and responsibly. It also provides a platform for children to ask questions and seek guidance when they encounter challenging online situations.

Conflict Resolution

Conflicts arising from social media-related issues, such as disagreements over screen time limits or concerns about online interactions, can strain family relationships. Open and honest communication is key to resolving these conflicts constructively. It enables family members to express their concerns, share their perspectives, and work together to find solutions that are mutually acceptable. Conflict resolution through dialogue helps prevent tensions from escalating and maintains a harmonious family environment.

Building Trust

Trust is a foundational element of healthy family relationships. When parents engage in open and honest conversations, they demonstrate trust in their children's ability to make responsible decisions. This trust, in turn, encourages children to confide in their parents and seek guidance when needed. Openness also involves transparency, where parents share their concerns, experiences, and perspectives with their children. This sharing of experiences helps children understand that their parents are partners in their digital journeys, ready to support and guide them.

Addressing the Impact of Social Media

Open and honest conversations should encompass a wide range of topics related to social media. It's essential to address both the positive and negative aspects to provide a balanced perspective. These conversations can cover areas such as:

Balancing Online and Offline

One of the primary challenges in the digital age is finding a balance between online and offline interactions. It's important to discuss the value of face-to-face communication and family time. Encourage children to recognize when excessive screen time is affecting their relationships and well-being. Teach them to self-regulate and disconnect from screens when necessary.

Setting Personal Boundaries

Children should understand the importance of setting personal boundaries in their online interactions. This includes knowing when to disconnect from screens, limit exposure to potentially harmful content, and prioritize real-world relationships. Parents can guide children in creating a healthy digital balance that aligns with their values and well-being.

Cyberbullying and Safety

Open conversations about online safety and cyberbullying prepare children to handle challenging situations. Parents can provide guidance on recognizing the signs of cyberbullying, responding appropriately, and seeking support when needed. Encourage children to share their online experiences, both positive and negative, to maintain open lines of communication.

Sharing Positive Experiences

In addition to discussing potential risks, parents should also create space for children to share positive online experiences. These can include connecting with distant relatives, learning new skills through online tutorials, participating in online communities that align with their interests, or using technology for educational purposes. By acknowledging the positive aspects of technology, parents can help children develop a balanced perspective.

REFLECTION AND GOAL SETTING FOR CONTINUED SUCCESS

Encouragement for Reflection

The Power of Reflection

Reflecting on one's actions and their outcomes is a powerful tool for personal growth and development. Encourage parents to take a moment to reflect on the positive changes they have initiated in their family's approach to social media usage.

This reflection can serve several important purposes:

Acknowledging Progress

Reflecting allows parents to acknowledge and celebrate the progress they have made in managing social media within their family. This celebration of small victories can boost morale and motivation.

Identifying Challenges

Reflection helps parents identify challenges they may have encountered along the way. By recognizing these challenges, parents can better address them in the future.

Understanding Impact

Parents can gain a deeper understanding of the impact their efforts have had on family dynamics, relationships, and the overall well-being of their children. This self-awareness is crucial for making informed decisions.

Positive Changes and Their Impact

It's essential for parents to consider the positive changes they have implemented. This could include setting screen time limits, promoting quality family time, or engaging in open conversations about social media. Parents can reflect on how these changes have influenced their family dynamics:

Improved Communication

Explore how open discussions about social media have improved communication within the family. Have children become more willing to share their experiences and concerns?

Stronger Bonds

Reflect on whether the quality time activities and shared experiences have strengthened the bonds between family members. Have these moments created lasting memories and deepened connections?

Screen Time Awareness

Consider whether the establishment of screen time limits has led to greater awareness among children about their screen usage. Have they become more mindful of their digital habits?

Acknowledging Successes and Areas for Improvement

Encourage parents to celebrate their successes, no matter how small. Whether it's a reduction in screen time, improved family communication, or the successful resolution of a social media-related issue, these achievements deserve recognition.

Highlight the importance of acknowledging the positive changes, as this can boost motivation and reinforce the idea that change is possible.

However, it's equally important to acknowledge areas for improvement. No strategy is perfect, and there may be aspects of social media management that still present challenges. Encourage parents to identify these areas and view them as opportunities for growth. By recognizing areas that require further attention, parents can continue to refine their approach to social media usage.

Goal Setting for Continued Success

The Role of Goal Setting

Goal setting is a dynamic process that plays a crucial role in sustaining positive changes. It provides direction, motivation, and a framework for continued growth. Parents can benefit from setting new goals that align with their family's evolving needs and the ever-changing landscape of technology.

Direction

Goals offer a clear sense of direction. They help parents identify where they want their family to be in terms of social media usage and family dynamics.

Motivation

Setting and achieving goals can be highly motivating. When parents have a clear vision of what they want to accomplish, they are more likely to stay committed to their efforts.

Framework for Improvement

Goals provide a structured framework for improvement. They break down larger objectives into smaller, manageable steps, making the process more achievable.

Practical Guidance on Goal Setting

Provide parents with practical guidance on setting new goals to enhance positive changes in social media usage. This guidance should encompass the following key aspects:

Identifying Specific Goals

Encourage parents to identify specific goals related to social media management. These could include reducing screen time during weekdays, improving the quality of family time, or further enhancing communication about online experiences.

SMART Goals

Emphasize the importance of SMART goals—goals that are Specific, Measurable, Achievable, Relevant, and Timebound. SMART goals provide clarity and structure. For example, a SMART goal could be: "Reduce screen time for each child to two hours on weekdays within the next three months."

Involving the Family

Goal setting should involve input from all family members. Parents can discuss goals with their children, seeking their input and buy-in. This collaborative approach ensures that goals are realistic and mutually beneficial.

Tracking Progress

Encourage parents to track their progress toward their goals. They can use various methods, such as keeping a journal, using screen time tracking apps, or conducting regular family meetings to assess how well they are meeting their objectives.

Flexibility and Adaptation

Stress the importance of flexibility in goal setting. Family needs and circumstances may change, as may the technological landscape. Parents should be prepared to adapt their goals as necessary to ensure they remain relevant and achievable.

Positive Reinforcement

Remind parents to celebrate milestones and achievements along the way. Positive reinforcement boosts motivation and encourages continued progress.

Nurturing a Culture of Reflection and Growth

Encouraging parents to engage in reflection and goal setting is essential for the sustained success of managing social media usage within families. Reflection allows parents to acknowledge progress, identify challenges, and understand the impact of their efforts. Celebrating successes and recognizing areas for improvement fosters motivation and growth. Goal setting, when approached thoughtfully and collaboratively, provides a clear path forward and ensures that positive changes continue to enhance family dynamics. By nurturing a culture of reflection and growth, parents can navigate the evolving digital landscape with confidence and ensure that their family remains at the center of their efforts.

11

REBUILDING TRUST AND CONNECTION

Examining the reasons behind the breakdown of trust

Trust is a fundamental component of any healthy relationship, and this holds true within the family unit. Parents inherently trust their children to make responsible choices, while children trust their parents to provide guidance and support. However, when social media addiction enters the picture, it can lead to a breakdown of trust due to several interconnected reasons:

Secrecy and Deception

One of the primary reasons behind the erosion of trust is the secrecy and deception that can accompany social media addiction. Adolescents and teenagers, in particular, may hide the extent of their social media use, leading parents to question their honesty. Trust is compromised when parents discover that their children have been concealing their online activities or engaging in risky behavior.

Loss of Control

Social media addiction can lead to a sense of powerlessness for both parents and children. Parents may feel that they have lost control over their child's screen time and online interactions, while children may perceive parental attempts to intervene as intrusive. This loss of control can erode trust as parents and children grapple with feelings of helplessness.

Impact on Responsibilities

As social media addiction consumes more of a child's time and attention, it often leads to a neglect of responsibilities such as schoolwork, chores, and family obligations. Parents may question their child's reliability and commitment to fulfilling their duties, which further erodes trust in the child's ability to balance their online and offline life.

Failed Promises

In some cases, children may make promises to reduce their social media use or address concerns raised by their parents. When these promises are consistently broken, it damages trust as parents perceive their child's inability or unwillingness to follow through on commitments.

Diminished Quality Time

Excessive screen time, driven by social media addiction, can result in a diminished quality of family time. When children prioritize their devices over spending time with their parents or engaging in family activities, parents may feel neglected and unimportant, contributing to the erosion of trust.

Negative Impact on Behavior

Social media addiction can lead to changes in a child's behavior, including irritability, mood swings, and withdrawal from family interactions. These changes can be distressing for parents, who may struggle to understand the underlying reasons for their child's altered behavior, leading to further mistrust.

Fear of Online Risks

Parents often worry about their child's online safety, including exposure to inappropriate content, cyberbullying, or online predators. When children do not communicate openly about their online experiences, parents may become increasingly concerned, leading to a breakdown in trust as they fear for their child's well-being.

Understanding these reasons behind the breakdown of trust is essential for parents seeking to rebuild their relationships with children affected by social media addiction. It highlights the complex dynamics at play and underscores the importance of addressing these issues openly and empathetically.

The role of communication breakdown and conflicts in eroding trust

Communication breakdown and conflicts play a pivotal role in the erosion of trust within parent-child relationships affected by social media addiction. Effective communication is the linchpin of trust, as it fosters understanding, empathy, and a sense of connection. However, when communication falters, mistrust can flourish. Here, we explore the specific ways in which communication breakdowns and conflicts contribute to the erosion of trust:

Lack of Transparency

Social media addiction often leads to a lack of transparency in parent-child relationships. Children may withhold information about their online activities, fearing parental judgment or consequences. This lack of openness stifles effective communication and prevents parents from fully understanding their child's online experiences.

Misunderstandings

Miscommunications and misunderstandings can arise when parents and children attempt to discuss social media addiction. Parents may perceive their child's behavior as rebellious or disrespectful, while children may feel that their parents do not understand the significance of their online connections. These misunderstandings can escalate into conflicts, further eroding trust.

Blame and Guilt

Conflicts related to social media addiction often lead to blame and guilt on both sides. Parents may blame their child for their excessive screen time, while children may feel blamed for causing distress within the family. These negative emotions can hinder effective communication and exacerbate the erosion of trust.

Unresolved Issues

When conflicts related to social media addiction remain unresolved, they can fester and intensify over time. Unaddressed issues can create a sense of frustration and hopelessness for both parents and children, making it challenging to rebuild trust.

Emotional Distance

Ongoing conflicts and communication breakdowns can result in emotional distance between parents and children. Parents may withdraw emotionally to protect themselves from further disappointment, while children may retreat into their online world as a coping mechanism. This emotional distance can deepen the mistrust between them.

Lack of Supportive Dialogue

In some cases, parents may resort to imposing rules and restrictions without engaging in supportive dialogue. This authoritarian approach can lead to power struggles and conflicts, making it difficult for children to trust their parents' intentions.

Failure to Address Root Causes

Effective communication should involve discussions about the underlying causes of social media addiction, such as stress, peer pressure, or emotional challenges. When these root causes remain unaddressed, conflicts tend to focus solely on symptoms rather than solutions.

To rebuild trust, parents must recognize the role that communication breakdowns and conflicts play in the erosion of trust. They should prioritize open, empathetic, and nonjudgmental communication with their children affected by social media addiction. Addressing these issues head-on is crucial for fostering understanding and ultimately rebuilding trust within the family.

STRATEGIES FOR REBUILDING TRUST

Rebuilding trust within parent-child relationships affected by social media addiction is a complex process that requires patience, understanding, and effective strategies. In this section, we delve into four key strategies for rebuilding trust and fostering healthier connections between parents and children:

Initiating open and non-judgmental conversations with children about their social media usage

Creating a Safe Space for Dialogue

The first step in rebuilding trust is to establish a safe and non-judgmental space for open conversations. Parents should convey to their children that they are willing to listen without criticism or immediate judgment. This creates an atmosphere where children feel comfortable sharing their thoughts, experiences, and concerns related to social media.

Active Listening

Active listening is a crucial component of open dialogue. Parents should practice active listening by giving their full attention, maintaining eye contact, and empathizing with their child's perspective. This validates the child's feelings and experiences, reinforcing the idea that their voice is heard and valued.

Avoiding Blame and Accusations

It's essential for parents to avoid placing blame or making accusations during these conversations. Instead, they should express their concerns using "I" statements, focusing on their feelings and observations rather than accusing the child. For example, saying,

"I've noticed you spend a lot of time on social media, and it worries me," is more constructive than, "You're always on your phone, and it's your fault."

Understanding the Child's Perspective

Rebuilding trust involves gaining a deeper understanding of the child's perspective. Parents should inquire about what they enjoy on social media, their online friendships, and any challenges they face. By showing genuine interest and empathy, parents can create a bridge of understanding between themselves and their child.

Exploring the Reasons Behind Social Media Usage

These conversations should delve into the underlying reasons behind the child's social media addiction. Children may use social media as an escape from stress, a means of connecting with friends, or a way to cope with emotional challenges. Understanding these motivations can guide parents in offering appropriate support and solutions.

Establishing clear boundaries and expectations regarding technology and online interactions

Collaborative Rule Setting

To rebuild trust and establish clear boundaries, parents should involve their children in the process of setting rules and expectations regarding technology use. This collaborative approach empowers children to take ownership of their online behavior and helps ensure that rules are realistic and acceptable to both parties.

Age-Appropriate Guidelines

It's crucial to consider age-appropriateness when setting boundaries. Younger children may require stricter limitations on screen time, while teenagers may benefit from more autonomy with defined boundaries. Parents should adapt rules to suit their child's developmental stage and maturity level.

Consistency and Enforcement

Establishing clear boundaries is only effective if they are consistently enforced. Parents should communicate consequences for violating these boundaries in a fair and consistent manner. This helps children understand the importance of adhering to the rules and reinforces the trustbuilding process.

Balancing Screen Time

A key aspect of setting boundaries involves striking a balance between screen time and other activities. Parents should encourage their children to engage in offline activities, such as sports, hobbies, and family interactions, to foster a balanced lifestyle.

Regular Check-Ins

It's essential for parents to conduct regular check-ins to assess how well the established boundaries are working. These check-ins provide opportunities to make adjustments based on the child's progress and any evolving needs.

Demonstrating consistent support and understanding to rebuild trust gradually

Patient Empowerment

Rebuilding trust is a gradual process, and parents must exhibit patience. Children affected by social media addiction often face challenges, and parents should empower them to make positive changes at their own pace. By offering consistent support, parents convey their commitment to the child's wellbeing.

Recognizing Efforts and Progress

Acknowledging and celebrating small achievements and efforts is essential. Parents should recognize and praise their child's steps toward healthier social media habits and offline engagement. This positive reinforcement encourages continued progress and builds trust.

Avoiding Criticism

It's crucial for parents to refrain from criticism or harsh judgments, even if setbacks occur. Criticism can hinder the trust-building process and lead to defensive reactions from the child. Instead, parents should offer constructive feedback and focus on solutions.

Being Reliable and Predictable

Children need reliability and predictability from their parents. Parents should strive to be consistent in their support, promises, and actions. When children can rely on their parents to be there for them, trust is reinforced.

Seeking professional guidance when necessary to facilitate the rebuilding process

Recognizing the Need for Professional Help

In some cases, social media addiction and the breakdown of trust may necessitate professional intervention. Parents should be open to the idea of seeking assistance from therapists, counselors, or addiction specialists when the challenges prove overwhelming.

Family Therapy

Family therapy can be a valuable resource for rebuilding

trust and improving parent-child relationships. Therapists can help facilitate communication, identify underlying issues, and guide the family toward healthier dynamics.

Individual Counseling

Individual counseling may be beneficial for both parents and children affected by social media addiction. It provides a space for each party to address their unique challenges and develop strategies for rebuilding trust.

Support Groups

Parents may find support groups for families dealing with social media addiction helpful. These groups provide a sense of community and shared experiences, offering emotional support and practical guidance.

Professional Guidance for Children

Children may benefit from individual counseling or support groups specifically tailored to address social media addiction.

These resources can help them develop healthier online habits and coping strategies.

FOSTERING CONNECTION

Rebuilding trust and connection within parent-child relationships affected by social media addiction is a journey that involves not only setting boundaries and rules but also actively nurturing the emotional bonds between parents and children. In this section, we delve into the importance of quality time, shared activities, and emotional connection as key components in rekindling and strengthening these vital relationships.

The importance of quality time and shared activities in rekindling parent-child connections

Quality Time as a Foundation

Quality time is the cornerstone of nurturing and rekindling parent-child connections. It involves dedicated, undistracted moments when parents and children can engage, connect, and create memories together. Quality time is essential for rebuilding trust and fostering a deeper understanding of each other.

Overcoming Digital Distractions

Social media addiction often leads to digital distractions that pull parents and children away from meaningful interactions. By intentionally setting aside time for each other without the intrusion of screens, families can work toward restoring the emotional bonds that may have been strained.

Shared Experiences

Shared activities and experiences provide opportunities for bonding that go beyond words. Engaging in activities together allows parents and children to connect on a deeper level, share laughter, and build positive memories. These shared experiences can create a sense of togetherness and strengthen the parent-child relationship.

Strategies for creating opportunities for bonding beyond screens

Family Rituals and Traditions

Establishing family rituals and traditions can be a powerful way to create opportunities for bonding. These can include weekly game nights, monthly outdoor adventures, or yearly family vacations. Consistently engaging in these activities fosters a sense of belonging and anticipation.

Tech-Free Zones

Designating specific areas in the home as tech-free zones can help reduce screen time and encourage face-to-face interactions. For example, the dining room can be a tech-free zone during family meals, allowing for meaningful conversations and connection.

Shared Hobbies

Identifying shared hobbies or interests within the family can be a great way to bond. Whether it's gardening, cooking, hiking, or crafting, engaging in activities that family members enjoy together promotes quality time and creates opportunities for mutual enjoyment.

Exploring Nature

Spending time outdoors and connecting with nature can be therapeutic and conducive to bonding. Outdoor activities like hiking, camping, or simply taking leisurely walks in a nearby park provide a chance for parents and children to connect away from screens.

Volunteer Work

Engaging in volunteer work as a family can instill a sense of purpose and togetherness. Volunteering fosters empathy, teaches valuable life lessons, and strengthens the family bond through shared experiences of giving back to the community.

Nurturing emotional connections through active listening and empathy

The Power of Active Listening

Active listening is a fundamental component of nurturing emotional connections. When parents actively listen to their children, they demonstrate empathy, validation, and a genuine interest in understanding their thoughts and feelings.

This fosters trust and encourages open communication.

Validation and Empathy

Parents should acknowledge and validate their child's emotions, even if they may not fully understand or agree with them. Expressing empathy and understanding creates a safe space for children to share their concerns, joys, and fears.

Non-Judgmental Environment

Creating a non-judgmental environment where children feel comfortable expressing themselves is crucial. Parents should refrain from criticizing or dismissing their child's emotions and opinions, allowing them to freely communicate without fear of judgment.

Encouraging Emotional Expression

Encouraging children to express their emotions, whether positive or negative, is vital for building emotional connections. Parents can ask open-ended questions and use prompts like "How did that make you feel?" to delve deeper into their child's emotional world.

Quality Conversations

Quality conversations involve meaningful dialogue that transcends surface-level topics. Parents should engage their children in conversations about their interests, dreams, fears, and aspirations. These conversations help parents understand their child's inner world and strengthen the emotional bond.

OVERCOMING CHALLENGES

Rebuilding trust and connection within parent-child relationships affected by social media addiction is a transformative journey, but it is not without its challenges. In this section, we delve into the various hurdles that parents may encounter, strategies for addressing resistance and setbacks, the importance of celebrating small victories, and the enduring commitment required to maintain strong parent-child relationships in the digital age.

Addressing resistance and setbacks in the trustbuilding process

Understanding Resistance

Resistance is a common response when parents attempt to set boundaries or address social media addiction. Children may resist change due to habit, peer pressure, or fear of missing out. Parents should recognize that resistance is a natural part of the process.

Effective Communication

To address resistance, parents must maintain open and effective communication. It's essential to validate the child's feelings and concerns while explaining the reasons behind the changes. Active listening, empathy, and patience are key components of overcoming resistance.

Negotiation and Compromise

In some cases, negotiation and compromise may be necessary to address resistance. Parents can involve their children in discussions about rules and consequences, allowing them to have a say in the process. This collaborative approach empowers children and encourages their cooperation.

Consistency

Consistency in enforcing boundaries is crucial to address resistance effectively. Parents must stand firm in their commitment to the established rules, even in the face of pushback. Over time, consistent enforcement helps children adapt to the new norms.

Seeking Professional Help

If resistance persists and becomes a significant obstacle, seeking professional help, such as family therapy or counseling, can provide additional support. Professionals can offer guidance on addressing underlying issues contributing to resistance.

Recognizing and celebrating small victories in rebuilding trust

The Power of Small Victories

Rebuilding trust is a gradual process that involves small steps and incremental changes. Recognizing and celebrating these small victories is essential for maintaining motivation and reinforcing positive behaviors.

Tracking Progress

Parents can track their child's progress in terms of reduced screen time, improved communication, or healthier online habits. Keeping a journal or using apps to monitor changes can serve as a visual representation of the journey.

Positive Reinforcement

Positive reinforcement, such as verbal praise, encouragement, or rewards, can be employed to celebrate small victories. When children demonstrate improved behavior or adherence to established rules, acknowledging and rewarding their efforts reinforces trust-building.

Family Celebrations

Setting aside specific moments for family celebrations of milestones and achievements can create a sense of unity and accomplishment. Family dinners, outings, or special activities can serve as occasions to celebrate together.

Emphasizing Effort

It's crucial to emphasize effort over perfection. Parents should acknowledge that setbacks and relapses may occur but that these moments are opportunities for growth and learning. The emphasis should be on the child's commitment to change.

The long-term commitment required to maintain strong parent-child relationships in the digital age

A Lifelong Journey

Maintaining strong parent-child relationships in the digital age is a lifelong commitment. As technology evolves and children grow, the challenges and dynamics will continually shift. Parents must remain adaptable and dedicated to the process.

Consistent Communication

Consistent and open communication should be an enduring aspect of the parent-child relationship. Regular checkins, discussions about online experiences, and sharing concerns are essential for staying connected.

Evolving Boundaries

As children mature, boundaries and rules must evolve to match their developmental stages. Parents should revisit and adjust boundaries to reflect their child's changing needs and responsibilities.

Role Modeling

Parents must continue to model healthy online behavior throughout their child's adolescence and beyond. Leading by example and demonstrating responsible tech use reinforces the importance of balance and mindfulness.

Staying Informed

Staying informed about the latest social media platforms, trends, and online risks is crucial. Parents should remain aware of the digital landscape to guide their children effectively and address emerging challenges.

Celebrating Milestones

Milestones in a child's life, such as birthdays, graduations, and achievements, provide opportunities to celebrate the enduring bond between parent and child. These moments reinforce the value of the relationship and the commitment to nurturing it.

12

BUILDING HEALTHY SCREEN TIME ROUTINES

In today's digital age, navigating the world of screens and devices is an integral part of parenting. As children grow and develop, their screen time needs and limitations evolve. In this chapter, we explore the significance of creating age-appropriate screen time schedules and provide practical guidelines for parents to establish daily and weekly routines that support their child's healthy development.

Identifying the specific screen time needs and limitations based on age and developmental stages

Understanding the developmental stages of children is fundamental to identifying their screen time needs and limitations. Here, we delve into the distinct characteristics and requirements of various age groups and how they relate to screen time:

Early Childhood (Ages 0-5)

- During early childhood, children are in the critical stage of brain development. Their screen time exposure should be minimal and focused on high-quality, educational content.
- Guidelines recommend no screen time for children under 18 months, except for video chats with family.
- For ages 2-5, screen time should be limited to one hour per day, emphasizing educational and age-appropriate programs.

Middle Childhood (Ages 6-12)

- As children enter middle childhood, they begin to engage with screens more extensively for educational purposes and entertainment.
- Screen time should be balanced with other activities, such as physical play, homework, and social interactions.
- Guidelines suggest 1-2 hours of recreational screen time per day, with an emphasis on content quality and parental guidance.

Adolescence (Ages 13-18)

- Adolescents are exposed to a wide range of digital devices and social media platforms.
- Parents should collaborate with their teenagers to establish responsible screen time habits, considering academic demands and extracurricular activities.
- Encouraging self-regulation and open communication is essential to address screen time challenges during adolescence.

Practical guidelines for setting daily and weekly screen time schedules

Creating effective screen time schedules involves striking a balance between productive screen use and other essential activities. Parents can implement the following practical guidelines to establish age-appropriate daily and weekly routines:

Setting Screen-Free Zones

Designate specific areas in the home, such as the dining room or bedrooms, as screen-free zones to encourage face-toface interactions and family bonding.

Consistency

Establish consistent screen time schedules, including designated hours for homework, recreational use, and devicefree times (e.g., during meals or before bedtime).

Homework and Learning

Prioritize screen time for educational purposes, such as completing homework assignments, conducting research, and engaging in educational apps or programs.

Outdoor Activities

Allocate time for outdoor activities, physical exercise, and sports to promote a healthy lifestyle and balance screen time with physical well-being.

Family Time

Dedicate regular slots for family time, including shared meals, outings, and game nights. These moments strengthen familial bonds and provide alternatives to screen-based entertainment.

Communication

Encourage open communication with children about their screen time preferences and interests. Collaboratively negotiate screen time schedules, taking into account academic responsibilities and extracurricular activities.

Media Literacy

Educate children about media literacy and critical thinking skills to help them navigate online content responsibly and discern between reliable and unreliable sources.

Monitoring and Parental Controls

Implement parental controls and monitoring tools to track screen time and ensure compliance with established schedules.

Flexibility

Maintain flexibility in screen time schedules to accommodate special occasions, holidays, and individual needs while staying within reasonable limits.

Review and Adaptation

Periodically review and adapt screen time schedules to reflect changes in a child's age, developmental stage, and evolving interests. Engage in discussions with older children and adolescents to collaboratively adjust routines.

INVOLVING CHILDREN IN RULE SETTING

Involving children in the process of establishing screen time routines is a crucial step in promoting responsible and balanced technology use. This chapter explores the significance of including children in these decisions and provides techniques for engaging them in discussions about screen time limits and rules.

The importance of involving children in the process of establishing screen time routines

Empowerment and Ownership

Involving children in setting screen time rules empowers them to take ownership of their digital habits. It encourages a sense of responsibility and accountability, teaching them valuable life skills.

Understanding and Collaboration

Children often have insights into their screen time needs and preferences. By including them in the decision-making process, parents gain a deeper understanding of their children's perspectives and can collaboratively work towards reasonable solutions.

Respect for Autonomy

As children grow and become more independent, respecting their autonomy is essential. Involving them in rule setting demonstrates respect for their growing autonomy while providing necessary guidance.

Educational Opportunity

The process of discussing screen time rules can be educational in itself. It offers parents an opportunity to teach children about responsible technology use, media literacy, and the importance of balance.

Conflict Reduction

When children have a say in the rules, it reduces the potential for conflicts related to screen time. They are more likely to adhere to guidelines they had a hand in creating.

Techniques for engaging children in discussions and decisions about screen time limits

Family Meetings

Schedule regular family meetings to discuss screen time rules and routines. These meetings provide a platform for open dialogue and shared decision-making.

Active Listening

Begin by actively listening to children's perspectives and concerns. Give them the opportunity to express their thoughts and feelings about screen time.

Collaborative Decision-Making

Involve children in decision-making processes by asking questions like, "How much screen time do you think is reasonable?" and "What activities would you like to prioritize besides screen time?"

Negotiation and Compromise

Encourage negotiation and compromise when necessary. If children request more screen time, discuss the conditions under which this can be granted, such as completing chores or homework.

Educational Discussions

Use discussions about screen time as educational opportunities. Share information about the potential effects of excessive screen time on health, sleep, and academic performance.

Setting Clear Expectations

Ensure that children understand the rules and expectations regarding screen time. Clear and concise guidelines help avoid confusion and disputes.

Visual Schedules

Create visual schedules or charts that outline daily routines, including screen time slots. Visual aids can be especially effective for younger children.

Reward Systems

Implement reward systems that recognize adherence to screen time rules. For instance, children can earn additional screen time by completing tasks or displaying responsible behavior.

Consistency and Flexibility

Maintain consistency in enforcing rules, but also be open to flexibility when warranted by special occasions or individual needs.

Regular Check-Ins

Schedule regular check-ins with children to assess their screen time habits and discuss any challenges or adjustments needed.

Model Responsible Behavior

Set an example by demonstrating responsible screen time habits yourself. Children are more likely to follow rules if they see their parents practicing what they preach.

Online Safety Education

Educate children about online safety, privacy, and the potential risks associated with screen time. Equip them with the knowledge to make informed decisions.

BALANCING SCREEN TIME WITH OTHER ACTIVITIES

Balancing screen time with a diverse range of other activities is essential for a well-rounded and healthy daily routine. In this section, we explore strategies for creating a balanced daily routine that includes schoolwork, family time, physical activity, and leisure while encouraging children to diversify their interests beyond screens.

Strategies for creating a balanced daily routine that includes schoolwork, family time, physical activity, and leisure

Prioritize Schoolwork

Allocate specific time slots for schoolwork and homework. Consistency in study routines enhances academic performance and ensures that screen time doesn't interfere with learning.

Family Time

Dedicate regular blocks of time for family activities and interactions. Family dinners, game nights, and outings promote bonding and create a screen-free environment.

Physical Activity

Schedule daily periods for physical activity. Encourage children to engage in sports, exercise, or outdoor play. Physical activity is crucial for physical health and helps offset sedentary screen time.

Creative and Leisure Activities

Include time for creative and leisure activities that don't involve screens. Art projects, reading, crafting, and hobbies offer alternatives for leisure and skill development.

Chores and Responsibilities

Assign age-appropriate chores and responsibilities to instill a sense of duty and contribute to the household. This also helps children understand the balance between leisure and responsibilities.

Relaxation and Wind-Down Time

Reserve time for relaxation and wind-down activities, especially in the evening. This promotes healthy sleep habits by reducing screen exposure before bedtime.

Flexible Scheduling

Maintain flexibility in scheduling to accommodate individual interests, extracurricular activities, and special occasions. Balance can be achieved through a combination of structured routines and adaptability.

Time Blocks

Use time blocking techniques to allocate specific time slots for different activities. For example, dedicate mornings to schoolwork, afternoons to physical activities, and evenings to family time and relaxation.

Visual Schedules

Create visual schedules or charts that outline the day's activities. Visual aids can help younger children understand and adhere to routines.

Tech-Free Zones

Designate certain areas of the home, such as bedrooms or the dining room, as tech-free zones during specific hours. This reinforces the importance of screen-free activities.

Encouraging children to diversify their interests beyond screens

Explore Interests

Encourage children to explore their interests and passions. Ask questions about their hobbies and talents, and support them in pursuing these activities.

Exposure to New Activities

Introduce children to new activities and experiences. Enroll them in classes or clubs that align with their interests, whether it's music, sports, art, or science.

Limit Passive Consumption

Encourage active engagement rather than passive screen time. Encourage children to create, build, or participate actively in their chosen activities.

Model Diversification

Be a role model by diversifying your own interests and hobbies beyond screens. Share your enthusiasm for reading, gardening, or other non-screen activities with your children.

Positive Reinforcement

Use positive reinforcement to reward children for engaging in non-screen activities. Offer praise and incentives for spending time on productive and creative endeavors.

Educational Content

Introduce educational content that aligns with your child's interests. For example, if they enjoy science fiction, provide books or activities related to science and technology.

Limit Screen Availability

Set limits on screen time availability, especially during the weekdays. When screens are less accessible, children are more likely to seek alternative activities.

Outdoor Exploration

Foster a love for the outdoors by going on nature hikes, camping trips, or exploring local parks. Outdoor experiences can captivate children's interest and provide a break from screens.

Peer Interaction

Encourage children to spend time with friends and peers in social activities that don't involve screens. Playdates, sports teams, and clubs promote healthy social connections.

Empower Decision-Making

Allow children to have a say in the activities they engage in outside of screens. When they have ownership over their choices, they are more likely to invest in their interests.

MONITORING AND ADJUSTING ROUTINES

Effective screen time routines require ongoing monitoring and the flexibility to adapt to changing needs and circumstances. In this section, we delve into the role of ongoing monitoring and assessment of screen time routines and provide strategies for adapting these routines to meet evolving requirements.

The role of ongoing monitoring and assessment of screen time routines

Continuous Evaluation

Regularly assess the effectiveness of the established screen time routines. Consider whether they align with the family's goals, whether children are adhering to the rules, and if screen time is balanced with other activities.

Feedback and Communication

Maintain open communication with children about their screen time experiences. Ask for their feedback on the established routines and whether they find them manageable and fair.

Tracking Usage

Utilize screen time tracking tools or apps to monitor how much time children spend on screens. These tools provide valuable data for assessing screen time habits.

Observation

Observe changes in children's behavior, mood, and academic performance. If screen time routines are affecting these areas negatively, it may indicate a need for adjustment.

Regular Family Check-Ins

Schedule regular family meetings to discuss screen time routines. These meetings offer an opportunity to share concerns, successes, and any necessary modifications.

Peer and School Feedback

Consider feedback from teachers and peers regarding children's screen time behavior. This external perspective can provide insights into potential issues.

Adjustment for Age and Development

Recognize that screen time needs evolve as children grow and their developmental stages change. What works for a young child may need adjustments for a teenager.

Stay Informed

Stay informed about the latest research on screen time and its effects on children's health and well-being. Updated knowledge can guide adjustments to routines.

Strategies for adapting routines to accommodate changing needs and circumstances

Flexible Guidelines

Keep screen time guidelines flexible and adaptable. Allow for adjustments when special circumstances arise, such as school vacations or family events.

Review and Revise

Regularly review screen time rules and revise them as needed. If certain rules are no longer effective or relevant, be willing to make changes.

Family Consensus

Engage children in discussions about routine adjustments. Seek their input on how routines can better align with their needs and interests.

Trial Periods

Implement trial periods for routine adjustments. This allows the family to test new rules before fully committing to them.

Gradual Changes

If significant changes are necessary, implement them gradually. Sudden and drastic adjustments may lead to resistance and conflicts.

Conflict Resolution

Address conflicts and concerns related to routine adjustments through open and respectful communication. Ensure that children understand the reasons for changes.

Setting Goals

Set specific goals for routine adjustments. Determine what outcomes you aim to achieve, such as improved academic performance, increased physical activity, or better family connections.

Support System

Involve other family members or caregivers in the adjustment process. A united front can help reinforce new routines.

Monitor the Impact

After making adjustments, closely monitor their impact on children's behavior and well-being. Assess whether the changes are achieving the desired outcomes.

Reinforce Positive Changes

Celebrate and reward positive changes resulting from routine adjustments. Positive reinforcement encourages children to adhere to the new rules.

Regular Review Cycles

Establish a regular schedule for reviewing and potentially revising screen time routines. This could be done quarterly or biannually to ensure that routines remain effective.

13
EMPOWERING PARENTS AND TEENS TOGETHER

BRIDGING THE GENERATION GAP

The generation gap between parents and tech-savvy teenagers is a prevalent and often challenging aspect of the digital age. In this section, we delve into the acknowledgment of this gap and emphasize the need for mutual respect and effective communication to bridge it.

Acknowledging the generation gap between parents and tech-savvy teenagers

The generation gap, a term that has been used for generations itself, refers to the differences in experiences, values, and perspectives between different age groups. In the context of the digital age, the gap is particularly pronounced when it comes to technology use. Here, we explore the various dimensions of this gap:

Technological Proficiency

Teenagers are often more proficient in using technology and navigating digital platforms than their parents. They grow up in a digital-native environment, while their parents may have adapted to technology later in life.

Digital Natives vs. Digital Immigrants

The generational gap is accentuated by the distinction between digital natives (teenagers) and digital immigrants (parents). Digital natives have grown up in a world where technology is seamlessly integrated into daily life, whereas digital immigrants have had to adapt to this new reality.

Rapid Technological Advancements

The pace of technological change is relentless. Teenagers are more adaptable to these rapid changes, while parents may find it challenging to keep up with the latest trends and innovations.

Communication Styles

Teenagers often prefer digital communication methods such as texting or social media, while parents may value faceto-face or phone conversations more. This difference in communication preferences can lead to misunderstandings.

Online Privacy and Safety

Parents may have heightened concerns about online privacy and safety, given their life experiences, while teenagers may be more inclined to share personal information online, sometimes without considering potential risks.

Screen Time Norms

What constitutes reasonable screen time varies between generations. Parents may have different expectations regarding screen time limits, content consumption, and appropriate online behavior.

Influence of Social Media

The role of social media in teenagers' lives can be a source of disconnect. While teenagers may rely heavily on social media for socializing and self-expression, parents may view it with skepticism or concern.

The need for mutual respect and communication to bridge this gap

Bridging the generation gap between parents and techsavvy teenagers is a crucial endeavor. It not only enhances the parent-child relationship but also fosters responsible technology use and digital citizenship. Here's how mutual respect and effective communication can facilitate this process:

Open Dialogue

Encourage open and non-judgmental dialogue between parents and teenagers. Create a safe space where both parties feel comfortable expressing their views and concerns.

Active Listening

Active listening is key to understanding each other's perspectives. Parents should genuinely listen to their teenagers, validating their experiences and feelings.

Empathy and Understanding

Empathize with the challenges each generation faces. Parents should recognize that growing up in a digital age presents unique pressures and opportunities for their teenagers.

Mutual Learning

Both parents and teenagers can learn from each other. Teenagers can impart technological knowledge to their parents, while parents can share life experiences and values.

Setting Boundaries Together

Collaboratively establish technology-related rules and boundaries. When both parties are involved in rule-setting, there's a greater sense of ownership and compliance.

Digital Literacy Education

Parents can play a role in educating their teenagers about digital literacy, online safety, and responsible technology use. This can be a bonding experience and a way to bridge the gap.

Shared Activities

Engage in shared activities that promote offline interactions and quality time. Activities such as family outings, hobbies, or sports can strengthen the parent-child bond.

Parental Role Modeling

Parents should model responsible technology use and digital etiquette. Teenagers are more likely to emulate their parents' behavior.

Respecting Privacy

While parents have a responsibility to ensure their teenagers' safety online, respecting their privacy is essential. Establish clear boundaries while also allowing for autonomy.

Stay Informed

Parents should make an effort to stay informed about the digital landscape. This demonstrates a willingness to engage with the changing technological world.

Seeking Common Ground

Identify common interests and activities that both parents and teenagers can enjoy. Finding shared hobbies or passions can bridge the generational gap.

Flexibility in Parenting

Recognize that parenting approaches need to adapt to the digital age. Flexibility in parenting styles and strategies can lead to better communication and understanding.

Bridging the generation gap between parents and techsavvy teenagers requires acknowledging differences, promoting mutual respect, and fostering open communication. When both generations actively engage with each other and the digital world, it paves the way for a more harmonious and informed family dynamic. Ultimately, it's about creating an environment where parents and teenagers learn from each other's experiences and navigate the digital age together.

EDUCATING TEENS ON RESPONSIBLE USAGE

As parents navigate the digital landscape alongside their tech-savvy teenagers, it becomes increasingly important to educate and empower young individuals to use social media responsibly. In this section, we explore various strategies for parents to guide their teenagers in responsible social media usage while fostering critical thinking skills and digital literacy.

Strategies for parents to educate their teenagers about responsible social media usage

Open and Honest Conversations

Communication is the cornerstone of responsible social media usage. Parents should initiate regular, open, and nonjudgmental conversations with their teenagers about their online experiences. This creates an environment where teenagers feel comfortable discussing challenges and concerns.

Setting Clear Expectations

Establish clear rules and expectations regarding social media usage. Clearly communicate the family's values, online etiquette, and safety guidelines. Involve teenagers in the rulesetting process to ensure their buy-in and understanding.

Lead by Example

Parents should model responsible social media behavior. Teenagers are more likely to emulate their parents' online conduct. Demonstrating positive digital citizenship sets a powerful example.

Digital Literacy Education

Actively educate teenagers about digital literacy. This includes teaching them to critically evaluate online content, recognize misinformation, and understand the consequences of their online actions. Encourage them to verify information from multiple sources.

Online Privacy and Security

Teach teenagers about online privacy and security. Emphasize the importance of strong, unique passwords, privacy settings, and the potential risks associated with sharing personal information online.

Balancing Screen Time

Discuss the importance of a balanced approach to technology use. Encourage teenagers to allocate time for offline activities, school-work, and in-person social interactions.

Cyberbullying Awareness

Raise awareness about cyberbullying and its impact. Encourage teenagers to report any instances of cyberbullying, whether they witness it or experience it themselves. Reinforce the importance of treating others with kindness and respect online.

Critical Thinking Skills

Foster critical thinking skills in teenagers. Teach them to question information, identify bias, and analyze the credibility of sources. Encourage them to think critically before sharing or reposting content.

Responsible Content Creation

If teenagers engage in content creation on social media, guide them on responsible content development. Discuss the potential consequences of sharing certain types of content and the importance of respecting intellectual property rights.

Digital Footprint Awareness

Help teenagers understand that their online actions leave a digital footprint. Discuss how their online presence can impact their future, including college admissions and employment opportunities.

Fostering critical thinking skills and digital literacy in teenagers

Media Literacy Education

Provide teenagers with media literacy education. Teach them to critically assess the media they consume, including news articles, videos, and advertisements. Encourage discussions about media bias and the role of media in society.

Source Evaluation

Teach teenagers how to evaluate the credibility of online sources. Discuss the importance of cross-referencing information and fact-checking before accepting it as truth.

Recognizing Manipulative Content

Help teenagers recognize manipulative content and persuasive techniques used in advertising and social media. Discuss the impact of algorithms and filter bubbles on the content they see.

Cybersecurity Awareness

Educate teenagers about cybersecurity best practices. This includes recognizing phishing attempts, protecting personal information, and using secure online practices.

Critical Reflection on Social Media Use

Encourage teenagers to reflect critically on their own social media use. Help them understand how the platforms may shape their behaviors and perceptions. Discuss the concept of the "highlight reel" on social media and its impact on self-esteem.

Dealing with Online Controversies

Guide teenagers on how to handle online controversies and polarizing discussions. Teach them strategies for engaging in respectful and constructive online conversations.

Digital Empathy and Compassion

Promote digital empathy and compassion. Encourage teenagers to consider the feelings and perspectives of others online. Discuss the potential consequences of cyberbullying and the importance of supporting peers.

Digital Activism and Social Responsibility

Explore the positive aspects of digital activism and social responsibility. Encourage teenagers to use social media as a platform for positive change and advocacy on issues they care about.

Encouraging Critical Reading

Encourage teenagers to read a variety of content from diverse sources. Promote critical reading habits and the exploration of different viewpoints.

Seeking Help and Guidance

Make sure teenagers know where to seek help or guidance if they encounter online content that makes them uncomfortable or if they witness harmful behavior. Create an environment where they feel safe discussing these experiences with trusted adults.

Educating teenagers on responsible social media usage, fostering critical thinking skills, and promoting digital literacy are essential components of preparing them to navigate the digital world responsibly and safely. Parents play a pivotal role in guiding their teenagers towards becoming responsible digital citizens who can critically evaluate, engage with, and contribute to the digital landscape in a positive and informed manner.

COLLABORATIVE DECISION-MAKING

In the modern digital age, it's crucial to involve teenagers in setting family rules and guidelines for social media usage. This collaborative approach not only empowers teenagers but also leads to more effective, respectful, and sustainable agreements. In this section, we will explore the advantages of involving teenagers in this process and discuss techniques for negotiating and reaching mutually agreeable decisions.

The advantages of involving teenagers in setting family rules and guidelines for social media usage

Ownership and Accountability

When teenagers actively participate in creating social media rules, they feel a sense of ownership and responsibility. They are more likely to adhere to rules they had a hand in shaping, as they recognize the fairness of those rules.

Respect and Trust

Involving teenagers in rule-setting demonstrates trust and respect for their opinions and abilities to make informed decisions. This fosters a positive parent-teenager relationship built on mutual respect.

Understanding of Consequences

Through active participation, teenagers gain a better understanding of the potential consequences of their online actions. They become more aware of the impact of their social media use on their lives and the lives of others.

Communication Skills

Collaborative decision-making promotes communication skills. Teenagers learn to express their thoughts, concerns, and ideas effectively, which is a valuable life skill.

Critical Thinking

Teenagers are encouraged to think critically about their social media habits and their impact. They develop the ability to question and evaluate the rationale behind rules and guidelines.

Conflict Resolution

Engaging in discussions about rules helps teenagers develop conflict resolution skills. They learn to negotiate, compromise, and find common ground—a valuable skill set for various aspects of life.

Adaptability and Flexibility

Teenagers who are part of the rule-setting process are more likely to adapt to changing circumstances and rules. They understand that rules may evolve as they grow and as technology changes.

Empowerment and Independence

Involvement in rule-setting empowers teenagers to take responsibility for their digital choices and actions. It fosters a sense of independence and self-regulation.

Holistic Perspective

Teenagers often have insights and perspectives that parents may not be aware of. Involving them ensures a more holistic approach to setting rules that consider both parent and teenager viewpoints.

Long-Term Commitment

Rules set collaboratively are more likely to be adhered to over the long term. Teenagers are less likely to rebel against rules they had a say in creating.

Techniques for negotiating and reaching mutually agreeable decisions

Active Listening

Parents should actively listen to their teenagers' thoughts and concerns about social media usage. This demonstrates respect and opens the door for productive dialogue.

Empathetic Communication

Empathy is crucial in understanding teenagers' perspectives. Parents should strive to see the world from their teenagers' point of view, acknowledging their unique challenges and experiences.

Brainstorming

Encourage brainstorming sessions where both parents and teenagers generate ideas for social media rules. This fosters creativity and inclusivity in the decision-making process.

Compromise

Teach teenagers the art of compromise. It's essential for them to understand that not all their preferences may be accommodated, but they can find middle ground.

Negotiation Skills

Adolescents should learn negotiation skills, such as effective communication, patience, and the ability to find mutually beneficial solutions.

Setting Clear Expectations

Ensure that both parties understand the expectations and consequences associated with the rules. Clarity is key to preventing misunderstandings.

Conflict Resolution Techniques

Teach teenagers conflict resolution techniques, such as "I statements" and active problem-solving. These skills can be valuable in all aspects of life.

Respectful Disagreement

Acknowledge that disagreements may occur, and that's okay. Encourage respectful disagreement, where both parties express their views without hostility.

Written Agreements

Consider formalizing the agreed-upon rules in a written agreement signed by both parents and teenagers. This document serves as a reference point and reinforces commitment.

Regular Review

Schedule regular reviews of the rules to ensure they remain relevant and effective. This allows for adjustments as teenagers grow and as the digital landscape evolves.

Involving teenagers in setting family rules and guidelines for social media usage yields numerous advantages, including ownership, trust, and improved communication. Techniques such as active listening, empathy, compromise, and negotiation are essential for reaching mutually agreeable decisions. This collaborative approach not only empowers teenagers but also strengthens the parent-teenager relationship and prepares teenagers for responsible decision-making in the digital age and beyond.

MAINTAINING OPEN COMMUNICATION

Effective communication is the cornerstone of healthy parent-teen relationships, especially in the context of social media usage. In this section, we will delve into the critical role of ongoing, open, and non-judgmental communication between parents and teenagers regarding social media. We will also explore strategies for encouraging teenagers to express their concerns and experiences.

The role of ongoing, open, and non-judgmental communication in parent-teen relationships

Building Trust and Connection

Ongoing communication fosters trust and strengthens the bond between parents and teenagers. When teenagers feel heard and understood, they are more likely to confide in their parents.

Understanding Teenagers' World

Open communication allows parents to gain insights into their teenagers' world, including their social media interactions, challenges, and experiences. This understanding is vital for effective guidance.

Empathy and Support

Parents who engage in open and non-judgmental communication convey empathy and support. Teenagers are more likely to seek help and guidance when they know their parents are there for them without judgment.

Conflict Resolution

Effective communication provides a platform for resolving conflicts and misunderstandings. It encourages healthy dialogue over disagreements and promotes peaceful resolutions.

Emotional Well-being

Discussing emotional well-being openly helps parents identify signs of stress, anxiety, or other issues related to social media.

Early intervention becomes possible when teenagers feel comfortable sharing their feelings.

Setting Expectations

Communication is essential for setting clear expectations regarding social media usage. When teenagers know the rules and consequences, they are more likely to adhere to them.

Guidance and Education

Parents can use open communication to educate teenagers about the potential risks and benefits of social media. It enables teenagers to make informed decisions.

Respect for Autonomy

Open communication respects teenagers' autonomy and independence. It acknowledges their growing maturity and their ability to make responsible choices.

Preventing Miscommunication

Miscommunication and misunderstandings can lead to conflicts. Open communication reduces the likelihood of miscommunication by allowing for clarification and context.

Strengthening Resilience

Honest discussions about challenges related to social media can help teenagers build resilience. They learn to navigate difficulties and make better choices in the digital world.

Encouraging teenagers to express their concerns and experiences regarding social media

Active Listening

Encourage teenagers to express themselves by actively listening to what they have to say. Show genuine interest in their thoughts, even if they differ from your own.

Create a Safe Space

Establish an environment where teenagers feel safe expressing their concerns without fear of punishment or judgment. Assure them that their opinions matter.

Ask Open-Ended Questions

Use open-ended questions to initiate conversations. These questions invite more detailed responses and encourage teenagers to share their experiences.

Respect Their Perspective

Respect that teenagers may have a different perspective on social media. Even if you disagree, acknowledge their viewpoint and validate their feelings.

Empathize with Their Challenges

Teenagers face unique challenges in the digital age. Empathize with these challenges, whether it's cyberbullying, peer pressure, or the fear of missing out (FOMO).

Normalize Sharing Experiences

Normalize the act of sharing experiences, both positive and negative. Let teenagers know that everyone encounters challenges on social media, and it's okay to seek guidance.

Use Real-Life Examples

Share real-life examples of your own experiences with social media or stories of others who have faced similar situations. These anecdotes can spark meaningful conversations.

Be Patient and Available

Patience is key when encouraging teenagers to open up. Be available for conversations when they are ready to talk, even if it's outside regular family time.

Avoid Lecturing

Avoid lecturing or giving unsolicited advice. Instead, offer guidance when they seek it. Lecturing can lead to resistance and closed communication.

Seek Feedback

Encourage feedback from teenagers about family rules and guidelines related to social media. Their input can lead to more effective and fair rules.

Ongoing, open, and non-judgmental communication is essential for nurturing healthy parent-teen relationships in the digital age. It builds trust, fosters understanding, and empowers teenagers to navigate the complexities of social media responsibly. Encouraging teenagers to express their concerns and experiences requires active listening, respect, empathy, and the creation of a safe space for dialogue. When parents and teenagers communicate openly, they can work together to make informed decisions about social media usage and strengthen their family bonds.

CONCLUSION

In an era characterized by the pervasive influence of screens and social media, the challenges of parenting have expanded into the digital realm, reshaping the dynamics between parents and teenagers. The overarching theme of our journey has been the quest for equilibrium - balancing the benefits of technology with the preservation of healthy, nurturing parentteen relationships. As we conclude this comprehensive exploration, it is abundantly clear that the path forward is illuminated by knowledge, empathy, and proactive strategies.

Our expedition began with the acknowledgment that social media addiction can corrode family bonds, particularly those between parents and their tech-immersed teenagers. We delved deep into recognizing the signs of addiction, understanding the behavioral indicators such as withdrawal symptoms, preoccupation, neglect of responsibilities, and the resultant negative consequences. Yet, we discovered that the road to recovery often necessitates profes- sional intervention, emphasizing the critical importance of seeking appropriate support from therapists, counselors, or support groups.

As we progressed through the chapters, we equipped ourselves with a repertoire of strategies aimed at reducing social media dependence and fostering open communication within families. Setting clear boundaries emerged as a fundamental tool, offering a practical means of defining and enforcing limits on screen time. Simultaneously, encouraging alternative activities beckoned children to explore interests beyond the digital realm, diversifying their experiences and reducing dependence on screens. The concept of digital detoxes emerged as a crucial element in resetting the balance of technology usage, providing practical tips for their implementation.

Open communication, as we discovered, was the cornerstone upon which trust and understanding were built. Parents were urged to engage in candid dialogues with their children, creating an environment that fostered open expression without judgment. By involving children in the rule-setting process, parents not only granted them a sense of agency but also opened channels for discussion. Engaging in shared activities and hobbies further strengthened familial bonds, bridging the gap between virtual and physical worlds.

The 7-Day Action Plan, presented as a structured approach to change, served as a beacon for many families. It allowed parents to assess current social media usage, establish clear house rules and consequences, communicate these boundaries to their children, and weave tech-free zones and quality bonding time into their daily routines. Active listening, open communication, and shared activities emerged as essential elements of the plan, guiding families toward trust, reconnection, and resilience.

Addressing challenges in the digital age, we uncovered strategies for handling resistance, managing peer pressure and social media influence, and supporting children in developing healthy digital habits. Parents were empowered to navigate the complexities of parenting in the digital era through effective communication techniques and educational efforts that nurtured critical thinking skills and digital literacy.

The chapter on parental resources further fortified our arsenal, providing a toolbox of recommended books, websites, apps, tools, local support groups, and counseling services. These resources have become invaluable assets for parents, offering expert guidance and practical solutions tailored to their specific needs.

Real-life experiences shared by parents provided relatable stories of triumphs and challenges. These testimonials illuminated the emotional and relational dimensions of social media addiction, offering insights into the resilience and determination exhibited by parents in overcoming obstacles. We learned that success could be achieved through setting boundaries, improving communication, seeking professional help, and celebrating small victories along the journey.

As we navigated "The Road Ahead," we discovered that sustaining positive changes in social media usage required ongoing effort, adaptability, and a commitment to nurturing meaningful connections within families. Strategies for making social media a healthy and balanced part of family life, reinforcing positive habits and boundaries, and prioritizing meaningful connections became guiding principles on this path.

Empowering parents and teens together, we acknowledged the generation gap and the importance of mutual respect and communication. Educating teens on responsible usage, collaborative decision-making, and maintaining open communication emerged as key strategies for fostering empowerment and understanding between parents and teenagers.

In building healthy screen time routines, we emphasized the significance of age-appropriate schedules, involving children in rule-setting, balancing screen time with other activities, and monitoring and adjusting routines. These practices serve as a foundation for responsible and mindful screen time usage within families.

In conclusion, our journey through the complexities of parenting in the digital age has underscored the resilience of families. By recognizing the challenges, seeking guidance, and implementing proactive strategies, parents can foster healthier relationships with their children, even in the face of social media addiction. The digital age need not be a barrier to connection; it can be a tool for building stronger, more meaningful bonds. With knowledge, empathy, and unwavering commitment, families can navigate the digital landscape together, reinforcing the values of trust, communication, and love in this evolving era.